Seafood Everyday

Delicious recipes from a country Tasmanian kitchen

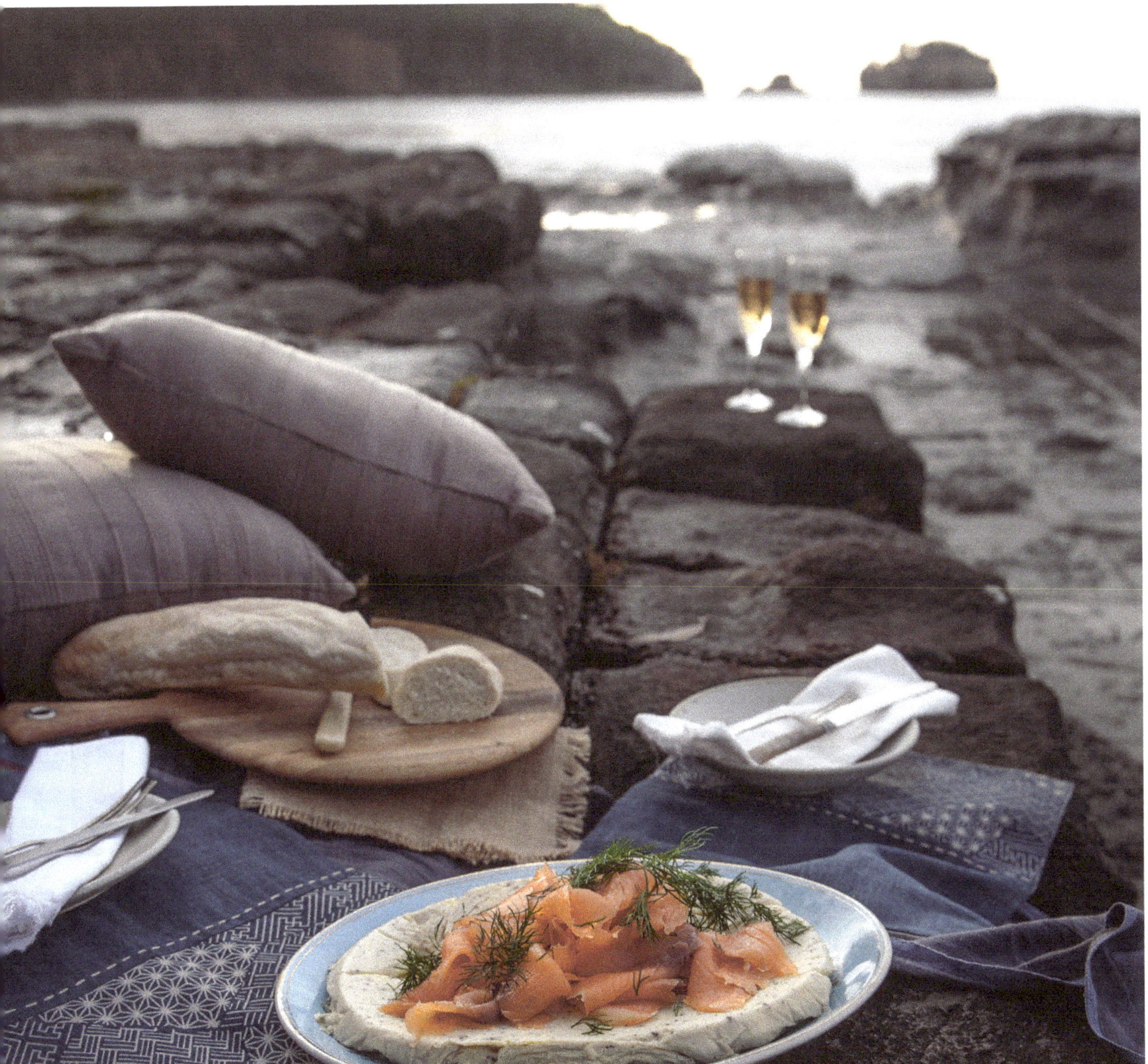

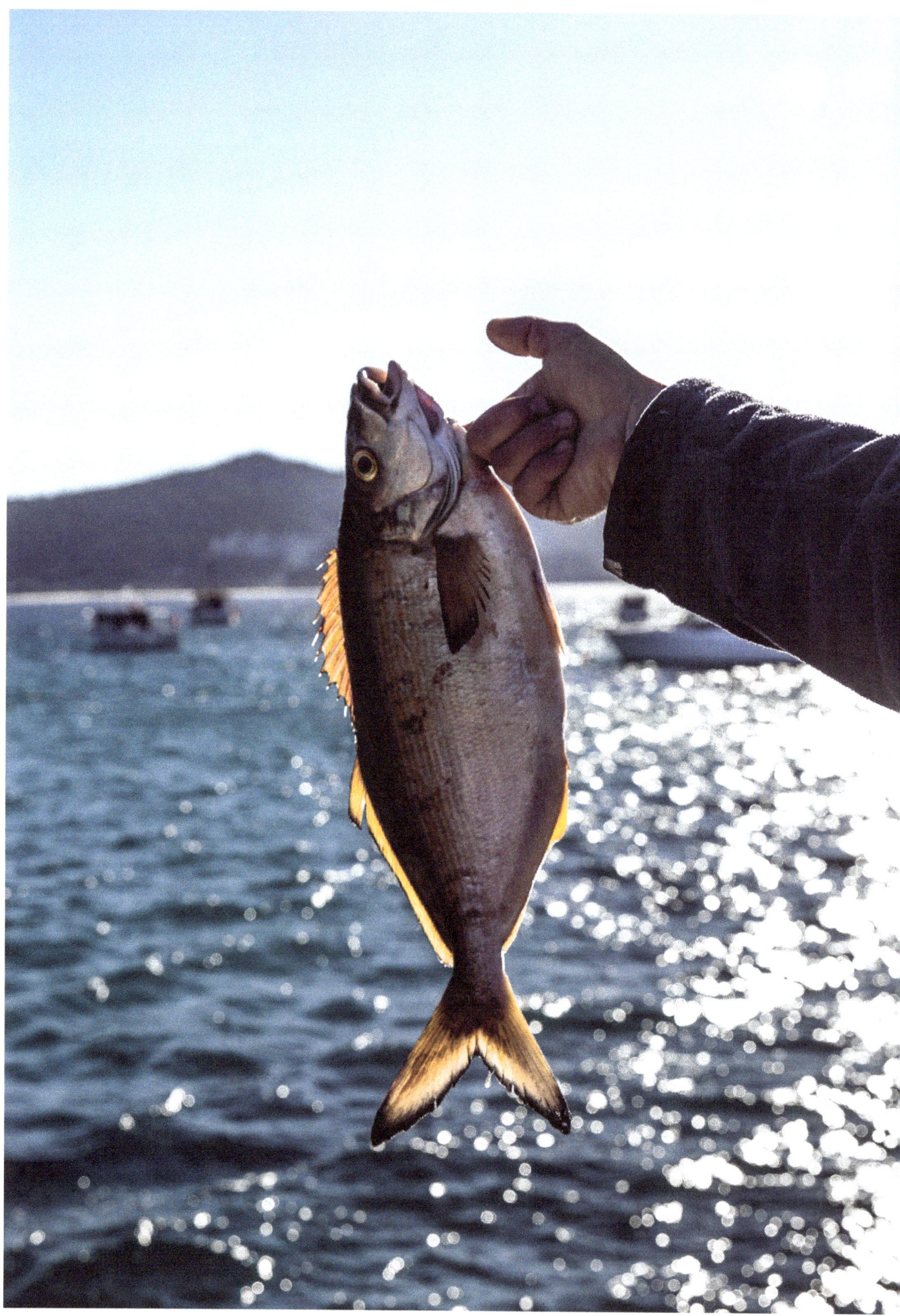

Seafood Everyday

Through varying sets of circumstances, I am the daughter, granddaughter and wife of a fisherman. With this ingrained fondness for the ocean, I really feel that producing a seafood cookbook was inevitable, one way or the other! For the last 15 years I have felt so fortunate to have lived on the Tasman Peninsula. Living and working in this wonderful place with my family provides us with the opportunity to catch, or collect, a wide variety of seafood from the surrounding waters. For seven years I was the chef and owner of my own popular, and highly acclaimed, restaurant at Taranna – The Mussel Boys. Over these years, it was common practice to have local fishermen dropping off bins of freshly caught fish at my back door, and we were able to collect oysters and mussels harvested, that moment, from local farms.

From a nutritional perspective, eating more fish and seafood is great for a healthy lifestyle, but one of the common complaints is that fish is too expensive. Yes, some of the higher-end, more popular fish that we see on restaurant menus is expensive, but there are also many, many more economical fish species that are commonly caught. Unfortunately, as many people don't know about cooking with these varieties, they don't sell so well at the fishmongers. As a result these cheaper species are commonly sold to other fishermen to use as bait for crayfish instead – but then who can afford crayfish for a weeknight family meal!? So, why not ask your fishmonger for a cheaper variety of fish, and let them know that you would buy it, if in stock. Finally, if you're not sure how to prepare or cook a less common variety of fish – just ask your fishmonger. They are always a wealth of knowledge. I also encourage everyone to feel more adventurous when cooking with squid, mussels and oysters as they are so readily available and nutritious.

It is important from both an economical sense, and a practical sense, that you select the right fish for each recipe. Spicy and strongly flavoured dishes don't need a delicate, expensive fish. You don't need to use a premium fish, such as flathead, to make spicy fish cakes or laksa. There are also plenty of meals that can be made with a good quality, well-frozen fish or quality tinned or smoked products.

We are so lucky in Tasmania to be able to source such high quality, fresh seafood. Just like with land-based farming, Tasmanian seafood is farmed to world's best practice, and we have a readily available and safe supply of mussels, oysters, salmon and other fish species. So, throw a line off the jetty, hook up the squid jig, take out the tinny or simply visit your local fish punts or fishmonger and start cooking with one of the best natural resources we have available to us, seafood.

I hope you enjoy these recipes for many years to come.

Eloise Emmett

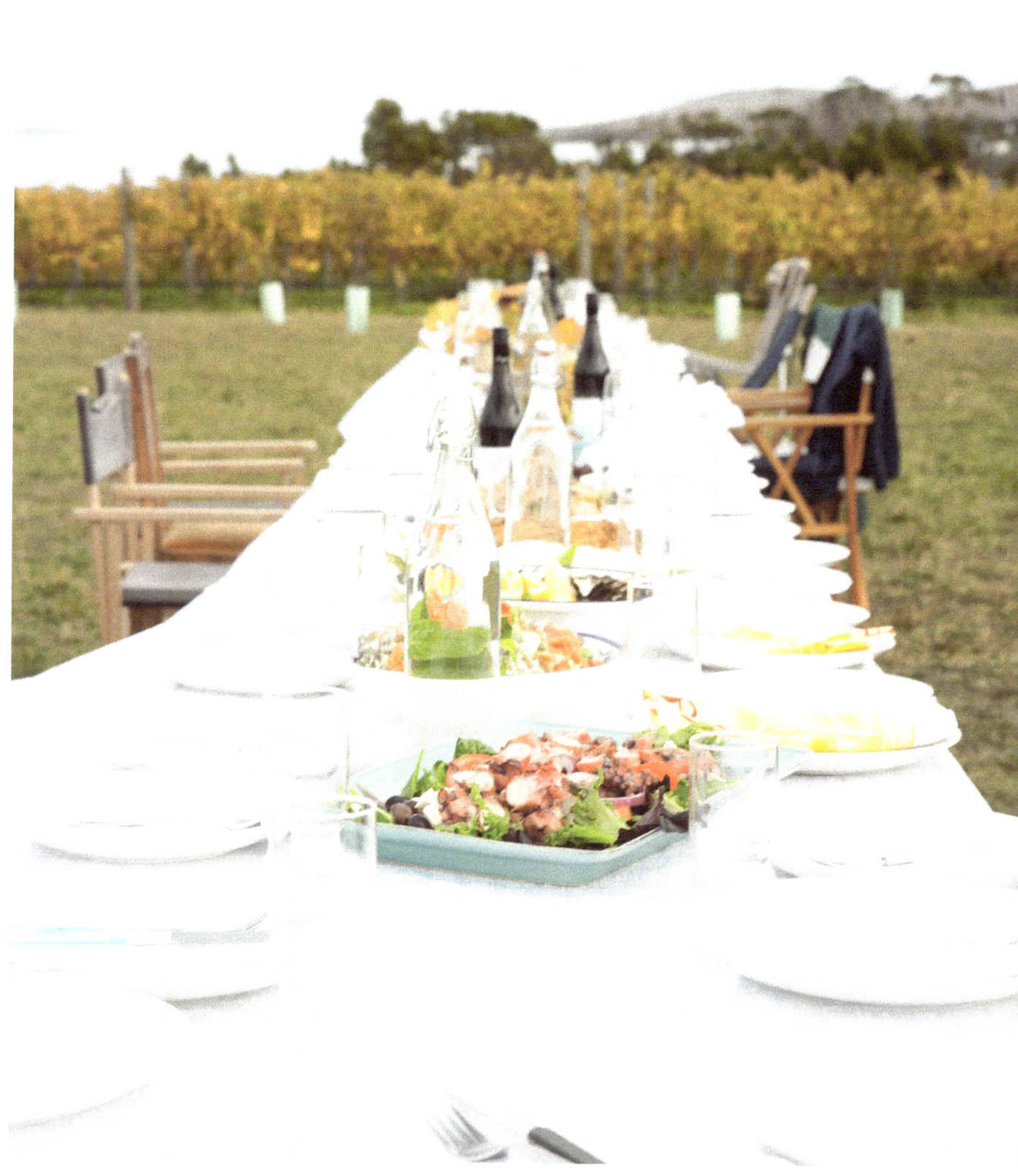

Acknowledgements

Thanks to all the readers of eloiseemmett.com, my cookbook owners, and Instagram and Facebook followers that inspire me to create new recipes regularly. A big thank you to my Workshop, Cooking Retreat and Indulgence Weekend guests at Little Norfolk Bay Events and Chalets for testing my new creations and inspiring me to create new recipes.

I would like to thank my family, my husband Brendan and children Maggie, Stephanie and Oscar for their support and patience while I take over our house for photo shoots and late nights in front of my computer editing recipes and photos.

Thanks to Kylie Berry, Stokely 9 Design, for the beautiful design and support with the creation of this book.

Thanks to Ian Wallace for the design work and project managing the production of the first edition of this book.

I would like to thank Katherine Burke and Sarah Carless for adding their lovely words to my recipes and editing the book.

Thanks to Lee-Anne Webb and Arwen Genge for cooking for the food photos.

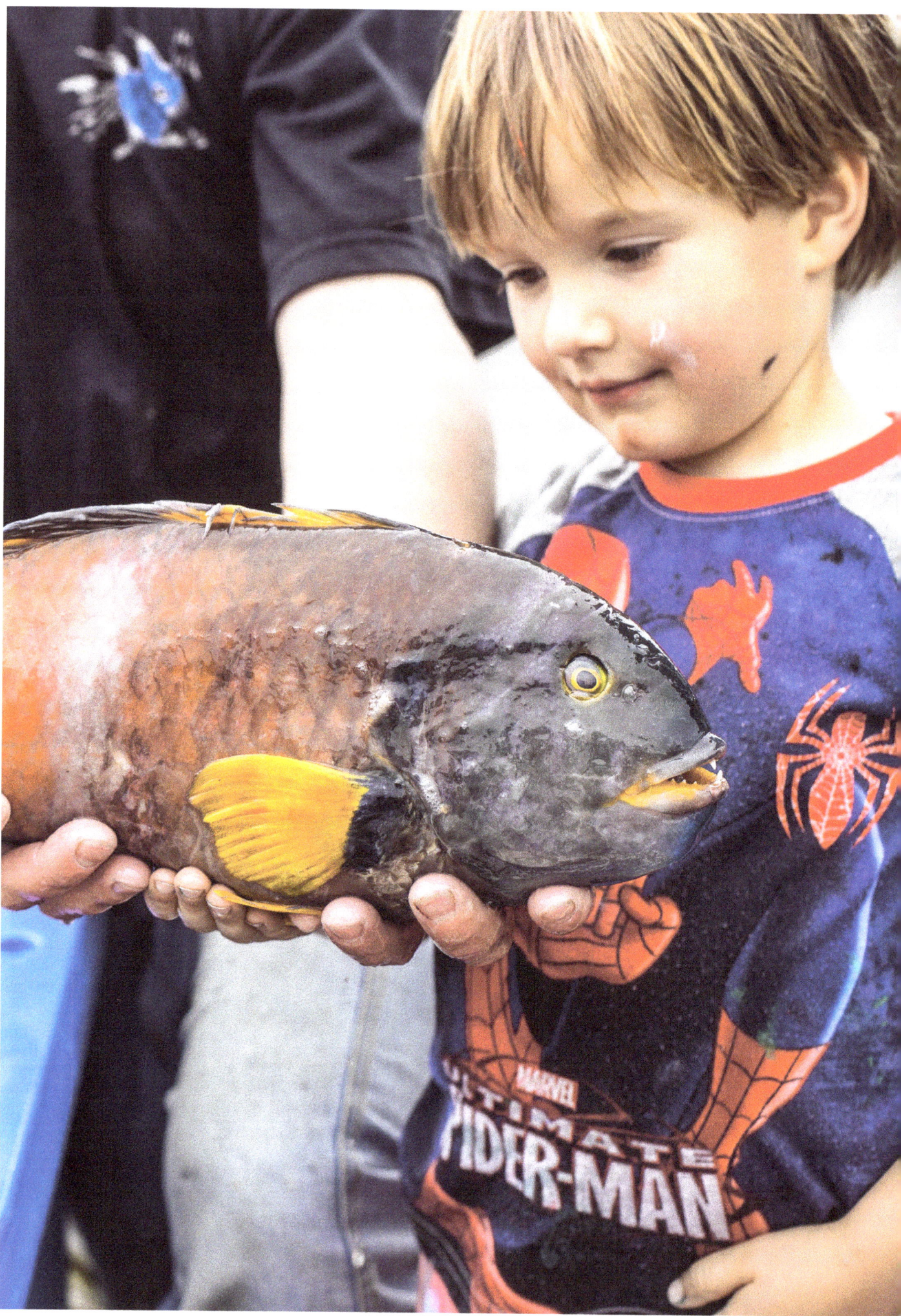

This book is divided into six chapters

SHELLFISH 8
Oyster, abalone and mussel dishes perfect as starters or for weeknight meals.

PANTRY STAPLES 38
Fish dishes from items you can have on hand in the cupboard or the freezer. Whilst fresh, local and organic is always best if you can get it, I'm not a food snob and I know that well preserved food such as frozen peas, spinach and canned fish are an economical and nutritious way to feed your family, especially in the off season.

ECONOMICAL FISH MEALS 60
These meals are delicious and with a bit of work and some additional flavour, are a good way to keep the family budget in check. Just like using cheaper cuts of beef, such as mince or stewing steak, these dishes often need a little extra cooking time or added flavour. Talk to your fishmonger, but fresh fillets of trevally, bay trumpeter, elephant fish, Australian Salmon are generally economical. Fresh fish is always best, but the recipes in this chapter will work well with frozen fillets. If you are lucky enough to catch your own fish, or find specials at the fish market, just pop them in the freezer for later use.

CEPHALOPODS 98
Octopus and squid are delicious and surprisingly easy to prepare. They are sometimes available at fishmongers, but your local seller will be likely to stock more if there is a demand, so be sure to ask. Unfortunately octopus can end up with other fisherman as bait, but it makes a wonderful seafood meal. Squid is also delicious and can also be an economical and popular family meal.

PREMIUM SPECIES 108
Popular and more expensive fish species such as Blue Eye Trevalla, Atlantic Salmon, Kingfish and Tuna are often seen at fish mongers and at restaurants for good reason – they are absolutely delicious! Just like using premium cuts of beef such as eye fillet, their high quality means that you really don't need to do much to create a delicious meal.

CRAYFISH 136
If you are lucky enough to catch or be given the occasional crayfish, these recipes in this chapter are wonderful for a special occasion, or you may choose to purchase a crayfish for a memorable meal.

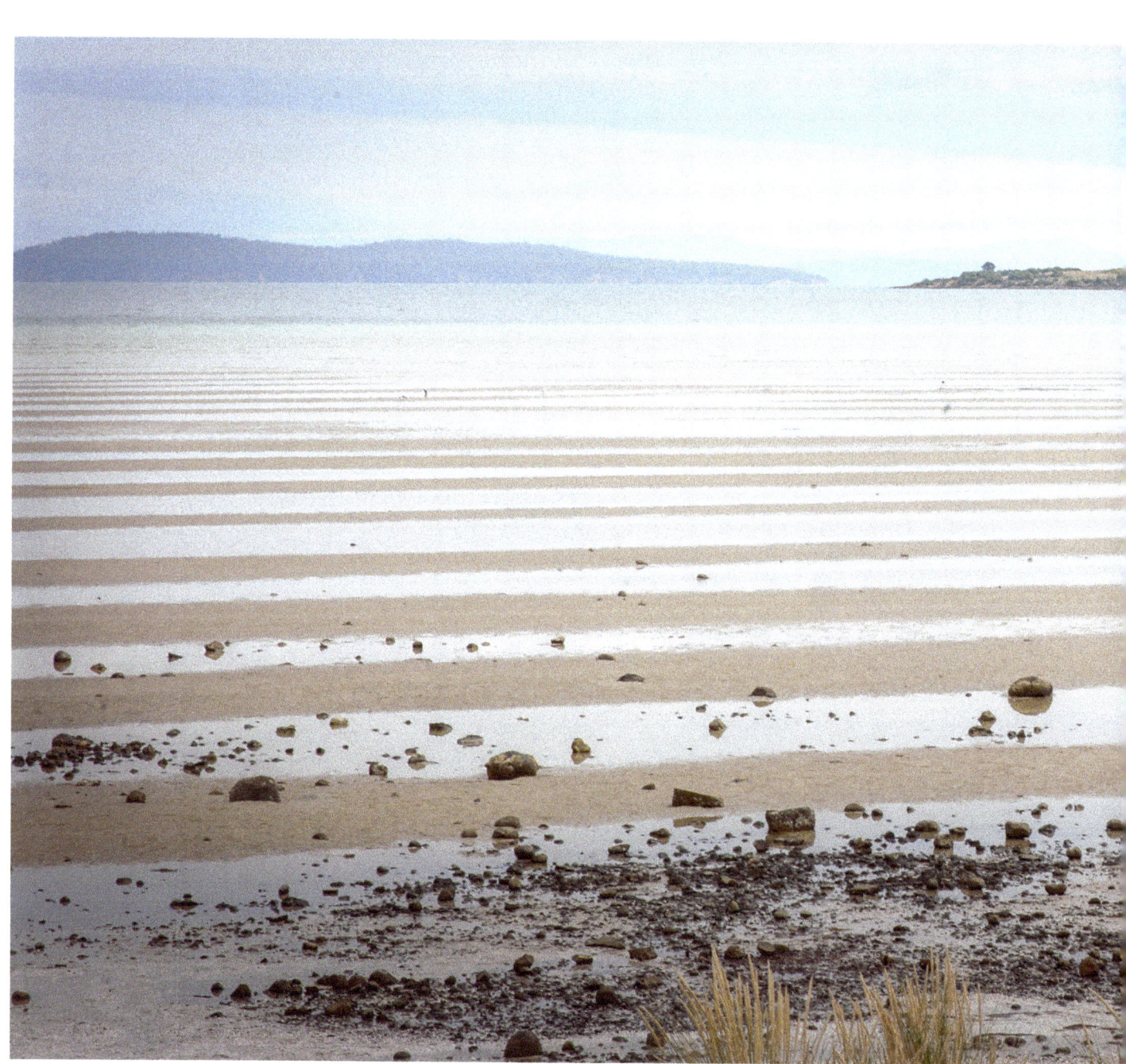

Shellfish

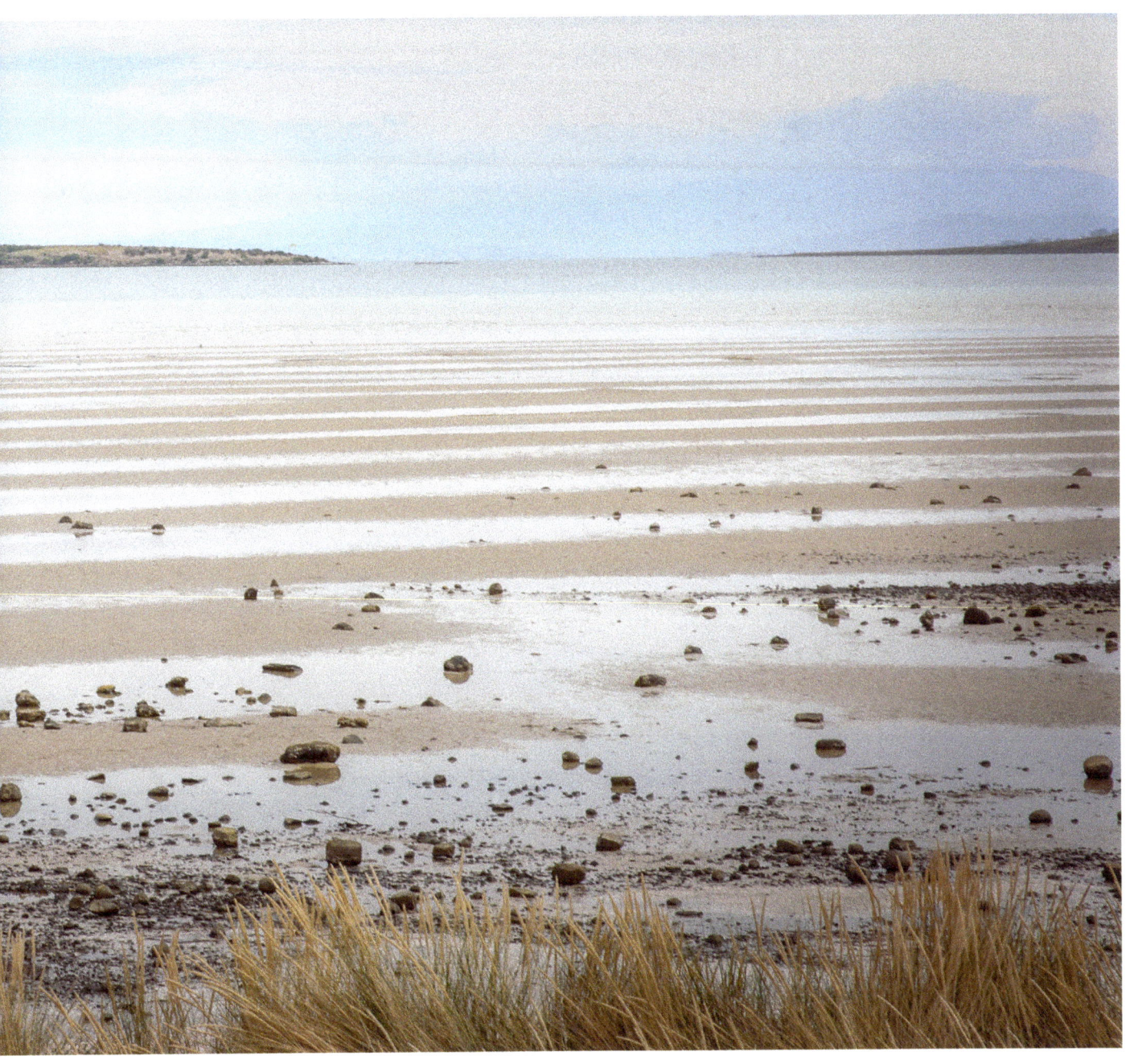

Salt and Sichuan Peppered Oysters

MAKES 1 DOZEN OYSTERS

½ cup plain flour

1 teaspoon salt

1 tablespoon ground Sichuan pepper

12 oysters in the half shell

1 tablespoon extra virgin olive oil

1 tablespoon butter

2 tablespoons sweet soy to serve

lemon and lime wedges to serve

Mix the flour, salt and pepper together in a bowl, or put them in a zip lock bag and shake to mix. Carefully remove the oysters from their shells. Roll the oysters in flour mix, or add to the bag and shake.

Heat the extra virgin olive oil and butter in a heavy based frying pan over moderate heat. Fry the oysters until golden brown on each side, or for about 1 minute.

Return the oysters to their shell for presentation if you wish and serve immediately with sweet soy sauce, lemon and lime wedges.

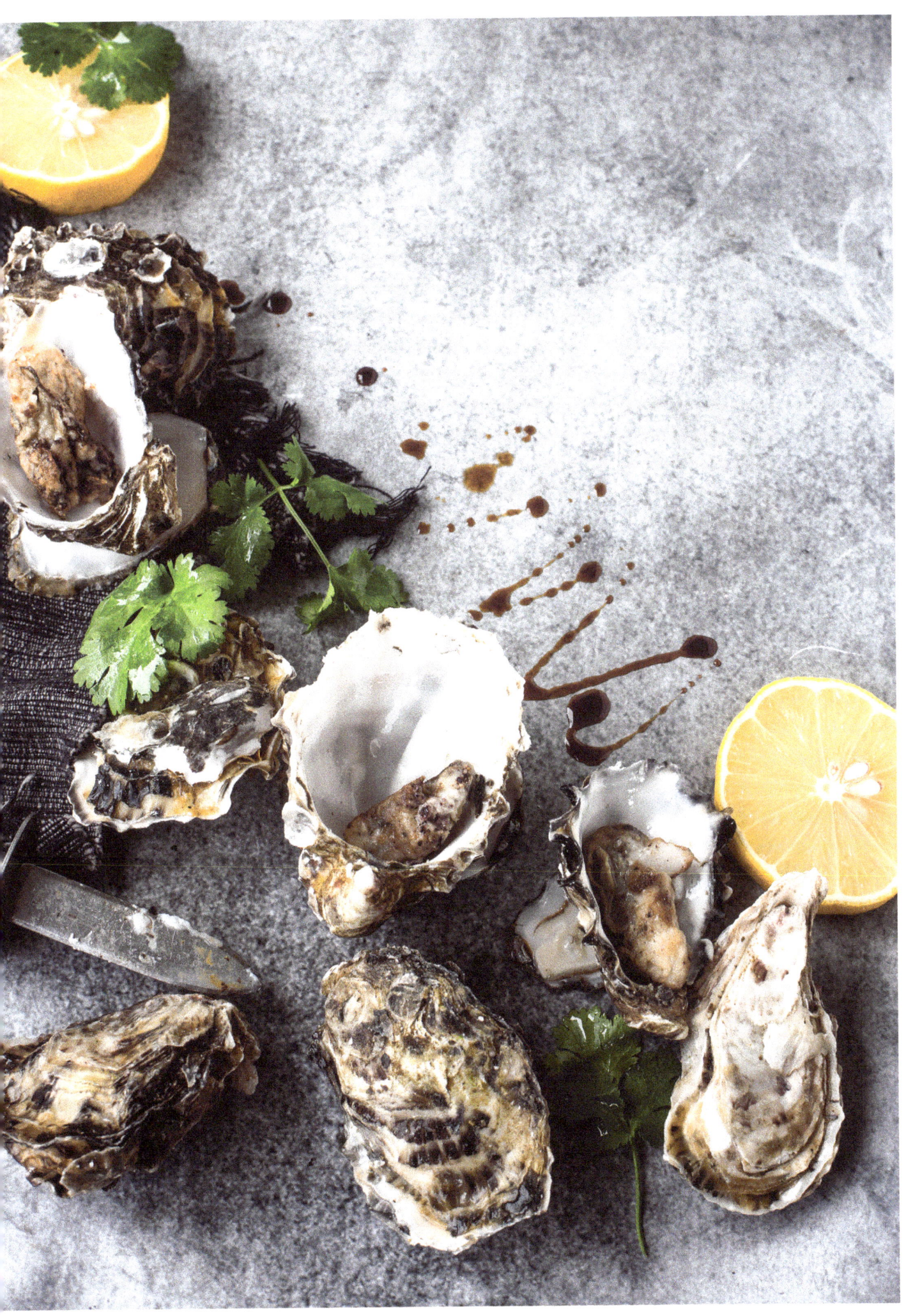

Oysters Florentine

MAKES 2 DOZEN OYSTERS

When making hollandaise sauce, the eggs yolks need to be whisked and lightly cooked. The best way to do this without scrambling the yolks is to cook over a saucepan of water. Just take care to select a bowl that fits tightly over the top of the saucepan.

24 oysters in the half shell

1 tablespoon butter for cooking oysters

100 grams English spinach

1 tablespoon butter

salt and pepper

HOLLANDAISE SAUCE

3 egg yolks

25ml white wine vinegar

150ml clarified (or melted) butter

salt and pepper

To make the hollandaise sauce, place the egg yolks and vinegar in a large bowl. Bring a saucepan of water to a simmer and place the bowl over the saucepan. Whisk the yolks and vinegar well, until the mixture becomes light and fluffy. While continuing to whisk, add the melted butter in a slow drizzle to create an emulsion. Season with salt and pepper.

The oysters can simply be warmed in the oven, or cooked if you prefer.

To warm the oysters, pre-heat the oven to 150°C. Place the oysters in their shells on a baking tray and warm in the oven for a few minutes.

To cook the oysters, remove the oysters from their shells. Place the shells in a 150°C oven to warm. Melt the butter in a frying pan over moderate heat, and sauté the oysters until just cooked. Return the oysters to their shells for presentation.

To cook the spinach, place a saucepan over medium heat and melt the butter. Add the spinach and sauté until wilted. Season with salt and pepper.

To serve top each oyster with the spinach and hollandaise sauce.

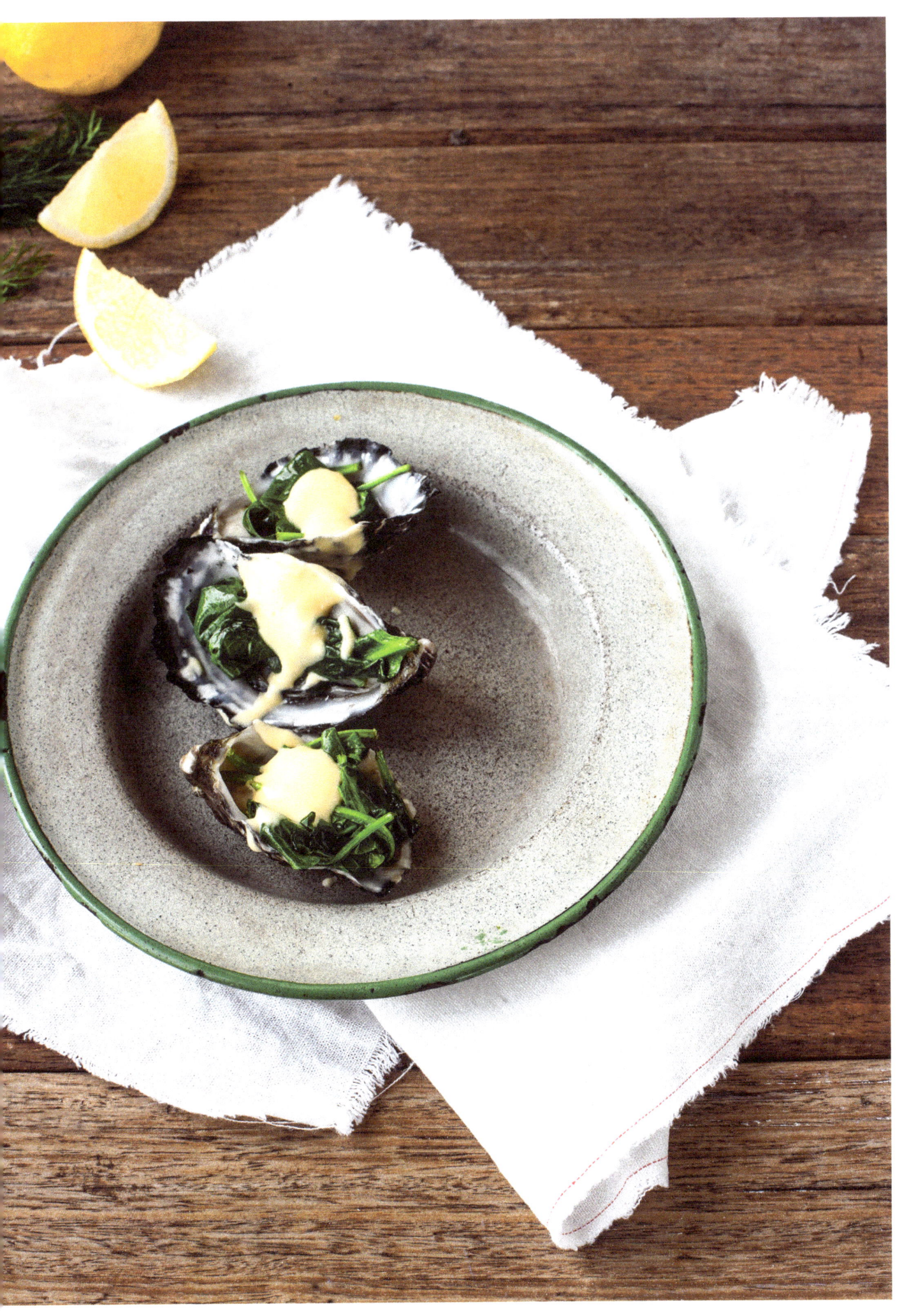

Oysters Grilled with Prosciutto and Gruyere

MAKES 1 DOZEN OYSTERS

12 oysters in the half shell

120 grams prosciutto

120 grams gruyere cheese

Pre-heat the grill to medium heat. Finely slice the prosciutto and thinly shave or grate the gruyere cheese. Top each oyster with the prosciutto and grill for 3 minutes or until the prosciutto is cooked. Top each oyster with cheese and grill for a further 2 minutes or until the cheese has melted. Serve immediately.

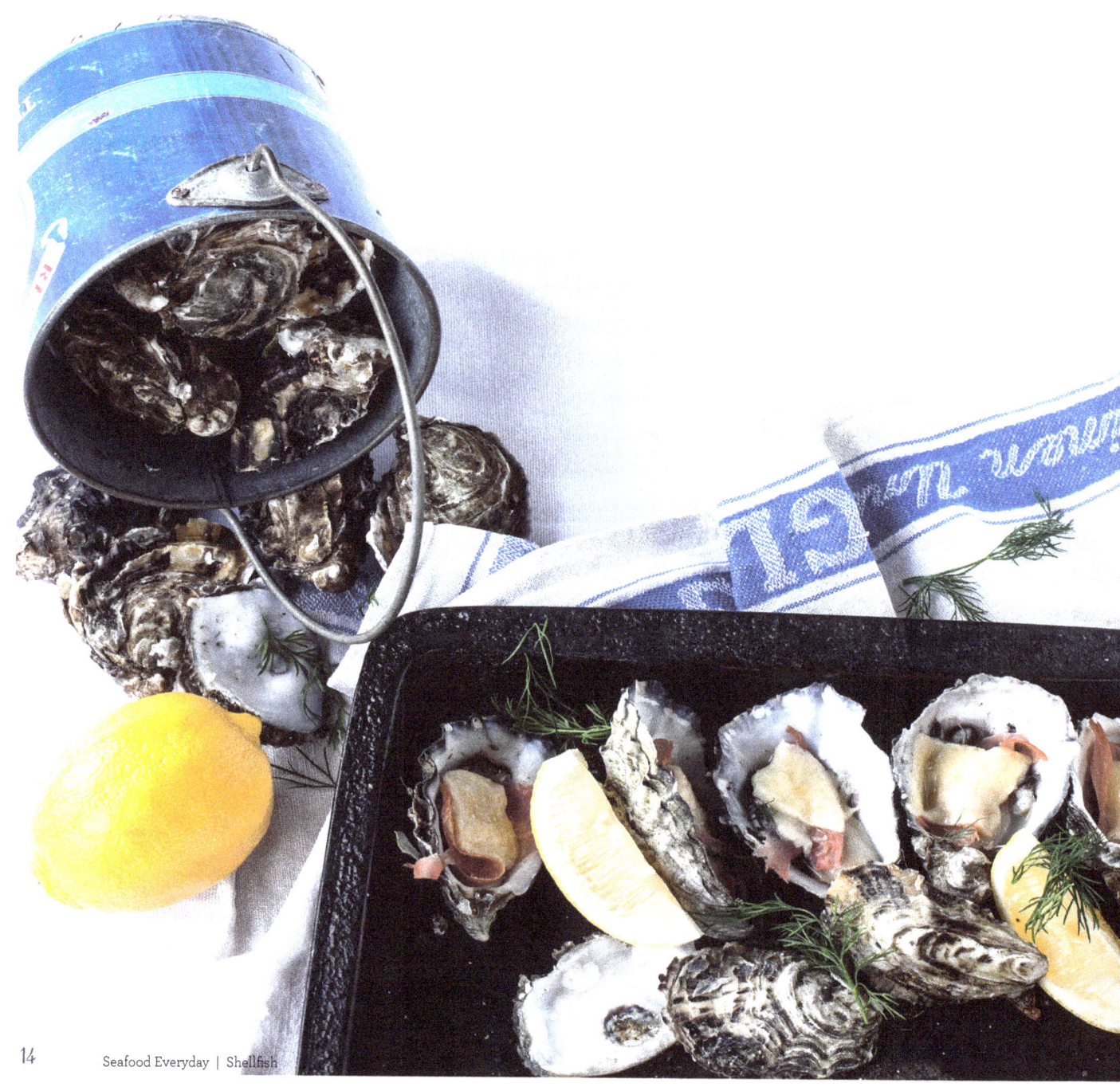

Oysters Topped with Tomato, Tabasco and Vodka Salsa

MAKES 1 DOZEN OYSTERS

2 vine-ripened tomatoes
2 large sprigs of dill
60ml vodka
Tabasco sauce
12 oysters in the half shell
lemon wedges to serve

Finely dice the tomato and finely chop the dill. Combine with the vodka and a splash of Tabasco sauce to your liking. Refrigerate this mixture for at least 15 minutes, but no longer than 4 hours (so that the tomatoes remain fresh). Top each oyster with the salsa and serve with lemon wedges.

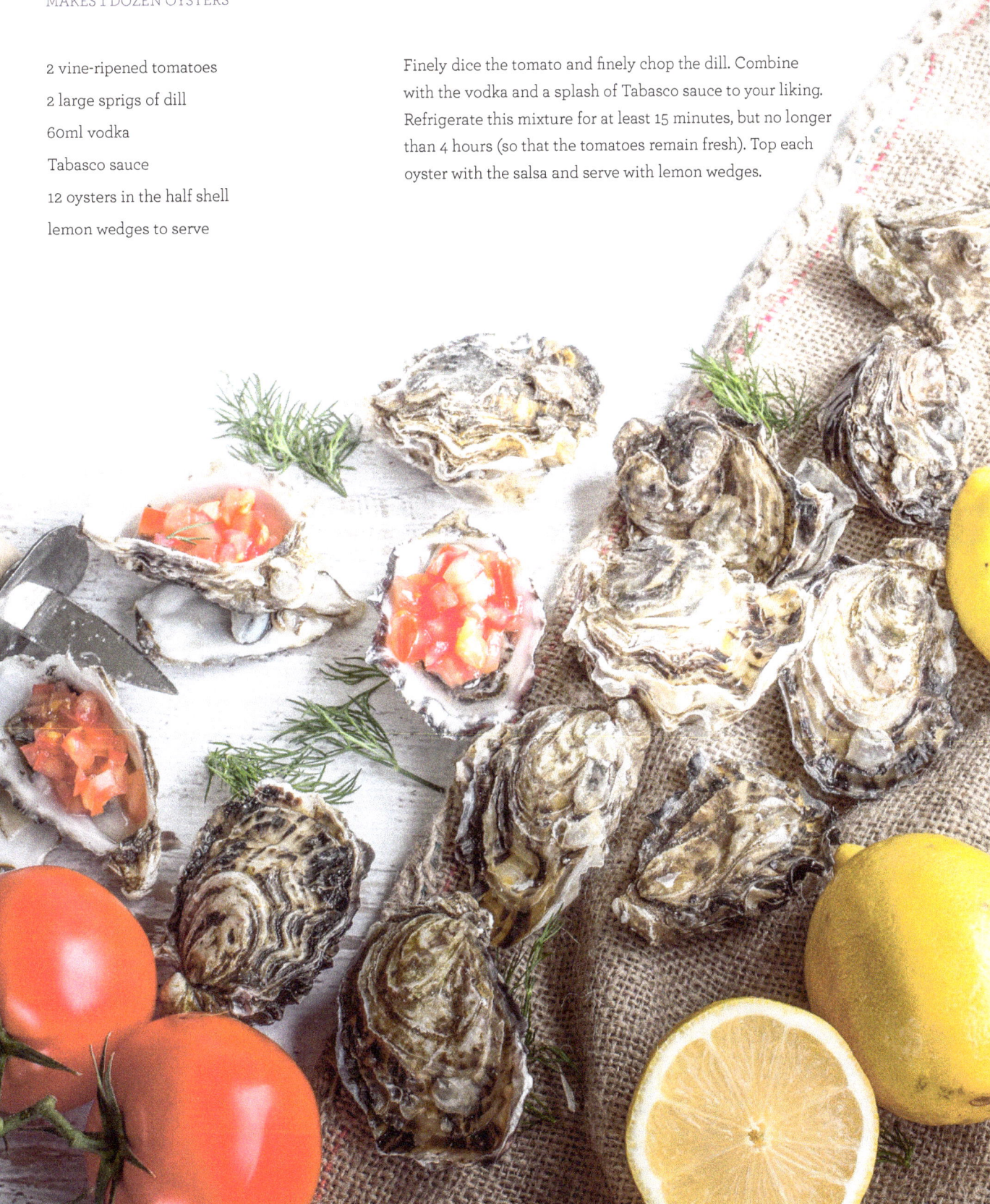

Oysters Topped with Smoked Salmon and Crème Fraiche

MAKES 1 DOZEN OYSTERS

120 grams smoked salmon

12 oysters in the half shell

120ml crème fraiche (or sour cream)

60 grams salmon pearls or roe

lemon wedges to serve

Finely chop the smoked salmon. Top each oyster with a tablespoon of smoked salmon, a teaspoon of crème fraiche and a sprinkle of the salmon pearls.

Serve immediately with the lemon wedges.

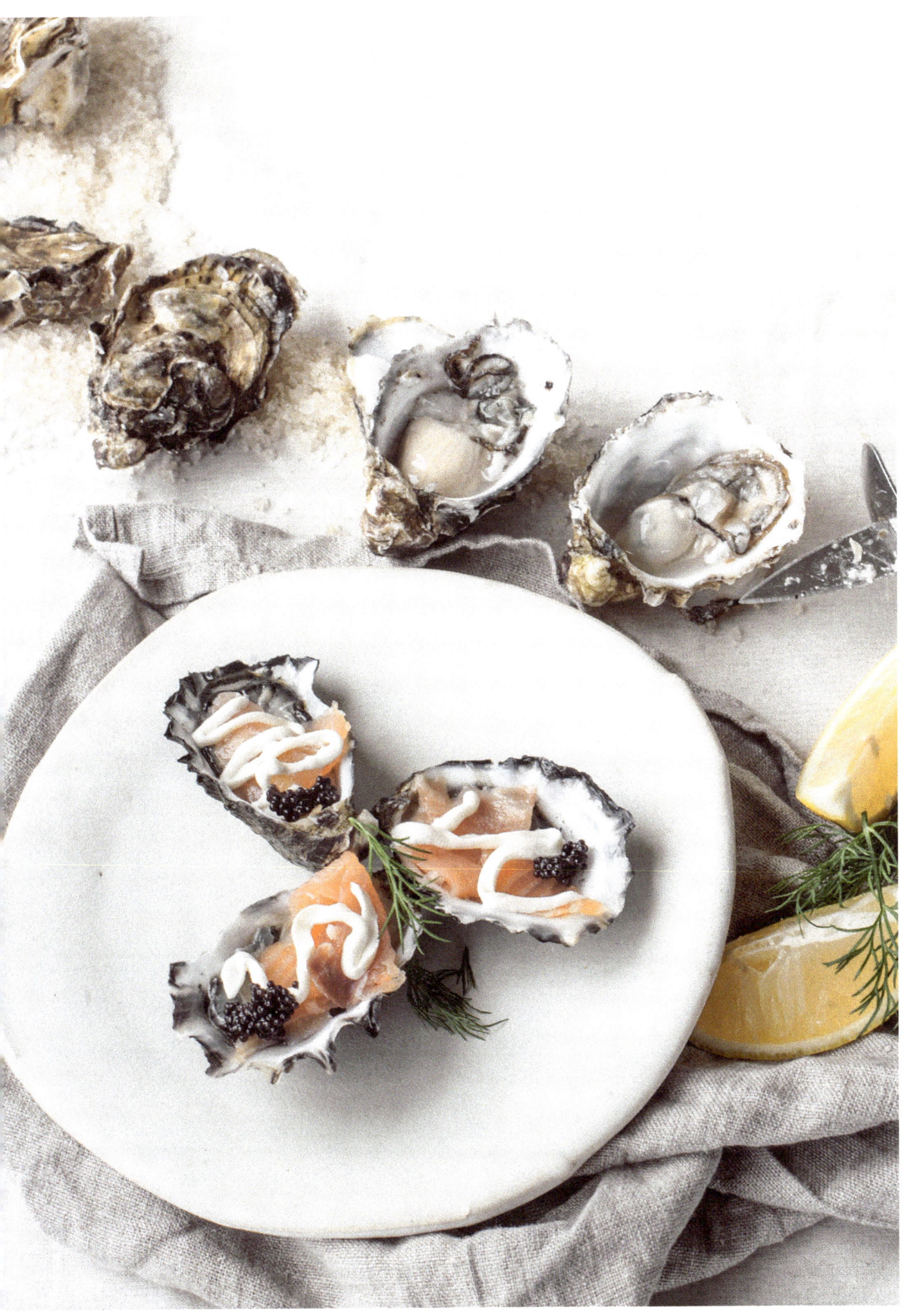

Oysters Topped with Red Wine Vinegar, Capers and Gherkin

MAKES 1 DOZEN OYSTERS

60 grams capers

60 grams gherkins

60ml red wine vinegar

12 oysters in the half shell

Finely chop the capers and gherkins and mix with the vinegar. Top each oyster with a spoonful of the mix and serve.

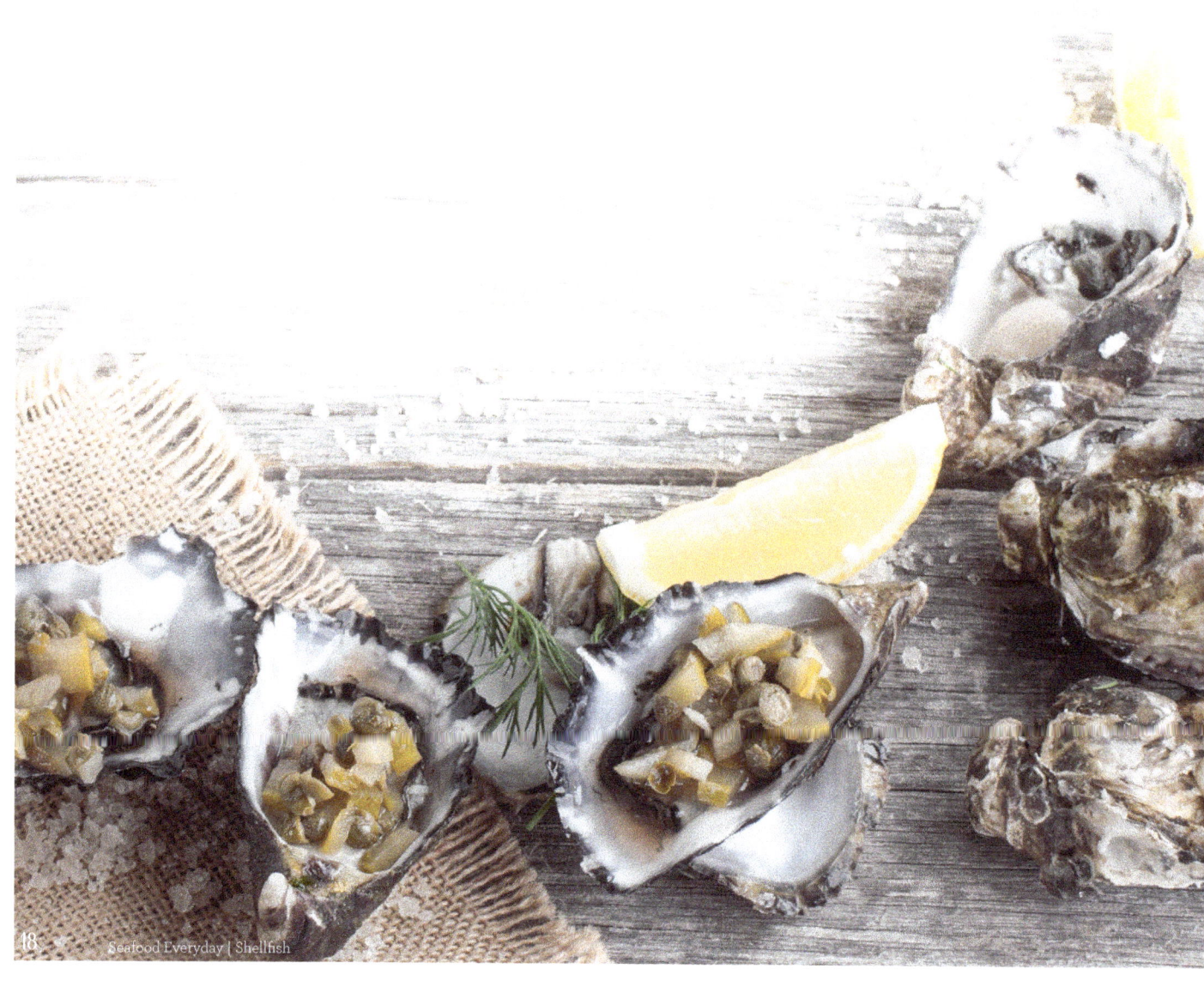

Natural Oysters with Lemon and Parsley Vinaigrette

MAKES 2 DOZEN OYSTERS

2 tablespoons parsley

1 tablespoon extra virgin olive oil

zest and juice of one lemon

1 teaspoon white wine vinegar

2 dozen natural oysters

To make the vinaigrette, finely chop the parsley and mix with the oil, lemon zest, lemon juice and vinegar.

Serve the vinaigrette as a dipping sauce for the oysters.

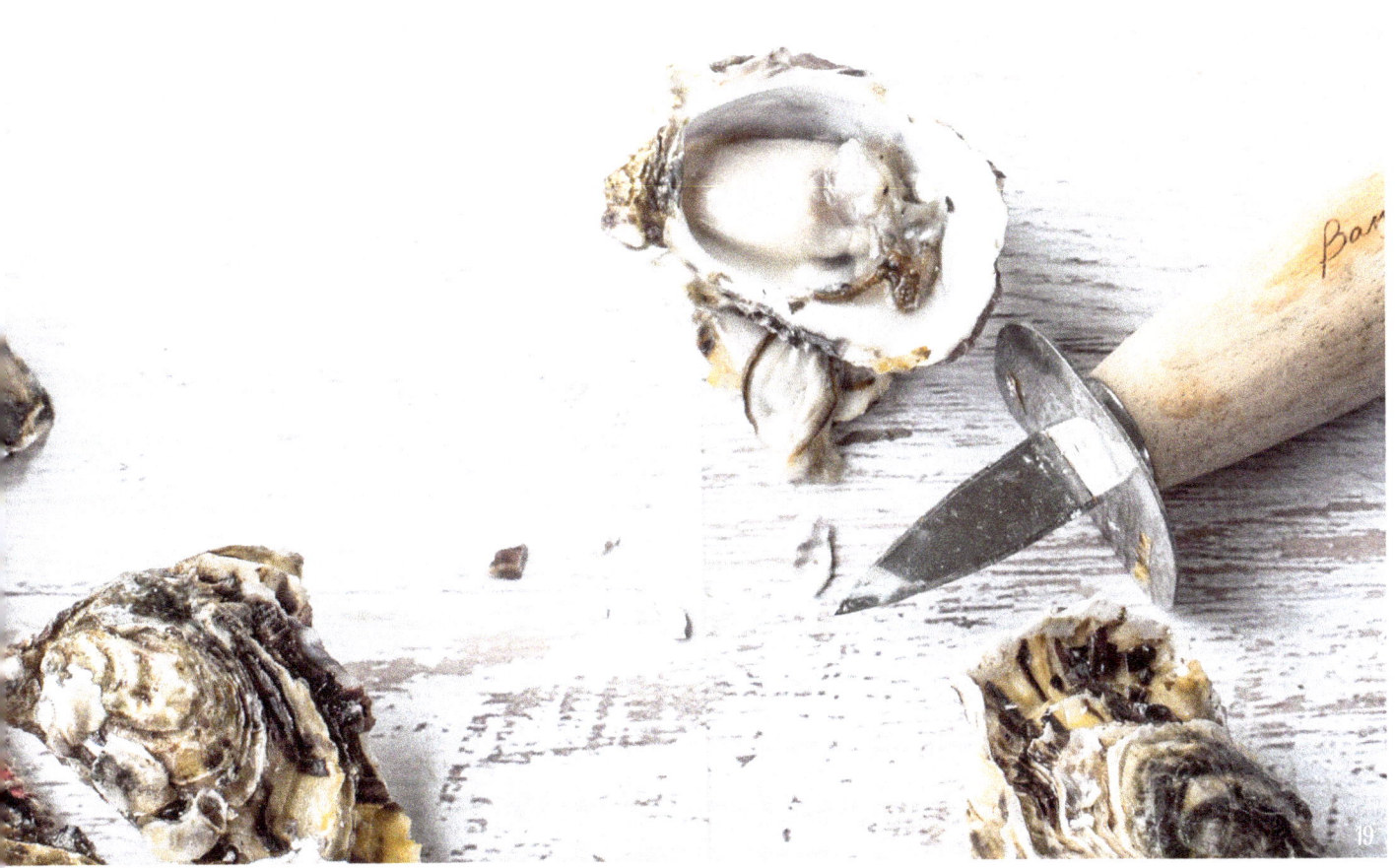

Tempura Oysters with Asian Dipping Sauce

MAKES 1 DOZEN OYSTERS

The Asian flavours in this dipping sauce taste best if you can make the sauce a day in advance to let the flavours develop.

DIPPING SAUCE

1 shallot

1 small red chili

1 clove garlic

2 tablespoons rice wine vinegar

1 ½ tablespoons fish sauce

1 tablespoon palm sugar

1 teaspoon lemon juice

TEMPURA OYSTERS

100 grams cornflour

100 grams self-raising flour

300ml soda water

2 tablespoons of plain flour

12 oysters in the half shell

extra virgin olive oil for deep frying

To make the dipping sauce, finely dice the shallot, finely chop the chili and crush the garlic. Mix with the rice wine vinegar, fish sauce, palm sugar and lemon juice. Refrigerate until required to let the flavours develop.

Heat the deep fryer to 180°C To make the tempura batter, combine the cornflour and self-raising flour in a bowl and whisk in the soda water. Put the plain flour on a plate and coat each oyster in the flour, then drop the oyster into the batter to coat. Deep fry the oysters until golden brown. Serve immediately with the dipping sauce.

If you don't have a deep fryer, you can deep fry the oysters in a saucepan of extra virgin olive oil filled at least 6cm deep. Heat the oil to 180°C before cooking.

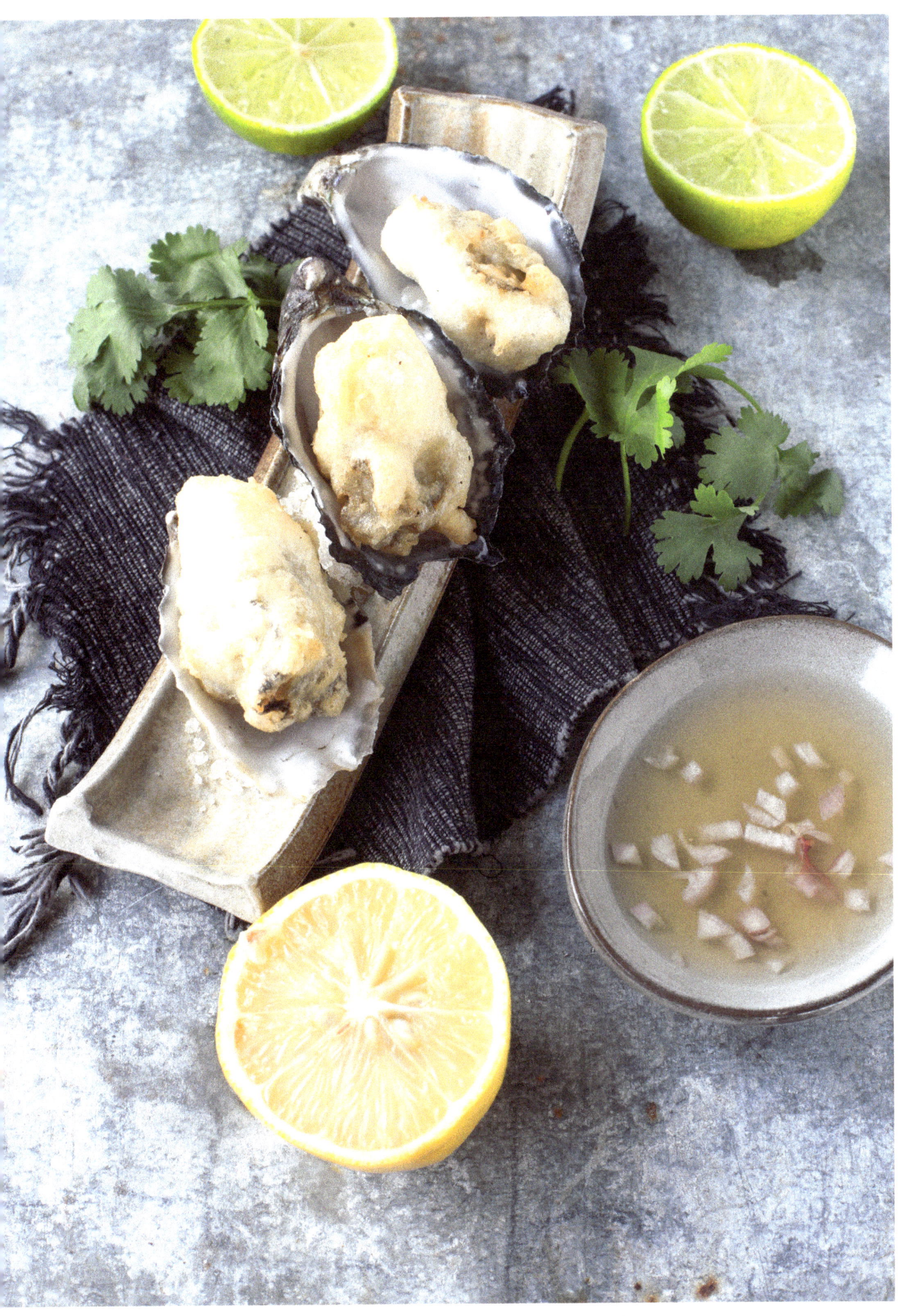

Scallops Wrapped in Bacon with Spicy Tomato Sauce

SERVES 4

This spicy tomato sauce can be cooked up to a couple of days in advance. For maximum deliciousness, leave the fat on the bacon in this dish. It is an important element in the cooking process of the scallops and the result is truly impressive.

400 gram scallop meat

400 grams bacon, sliced thinly

TOMATO AND CHILLI SAUCE

½ onion

3 large garlic cloves

2 birds eye chillies

1 tablespoon basil

1 tablespoon oregano

25ml extra virgin olive oil

400 grams crushed tomatoes

100ml white wine

To make the tomato sauce, chop the onion, crush the garlic and chillies, and chop the herbs. Heat the extra virgin olive oil in a large heavy-based pan over low heat, and sweat the onion, garlic, and chillies
until soft. Add the tomatoes and herbs and simmer gently for 15 minutes.

To prepare the scallops, slice the bacon in long pieces, approximately 2 cm wide. Wrap each piece around a scallop and push onto a skewer.

To cook the scallops, heat a frying pan or flat barbeque grill to medium-hot. Cook the scallops, turning regularly until the bacon is brown and crispy, and the scallops are cooked. Serve immediately with the hot tomato and chilli sauce.

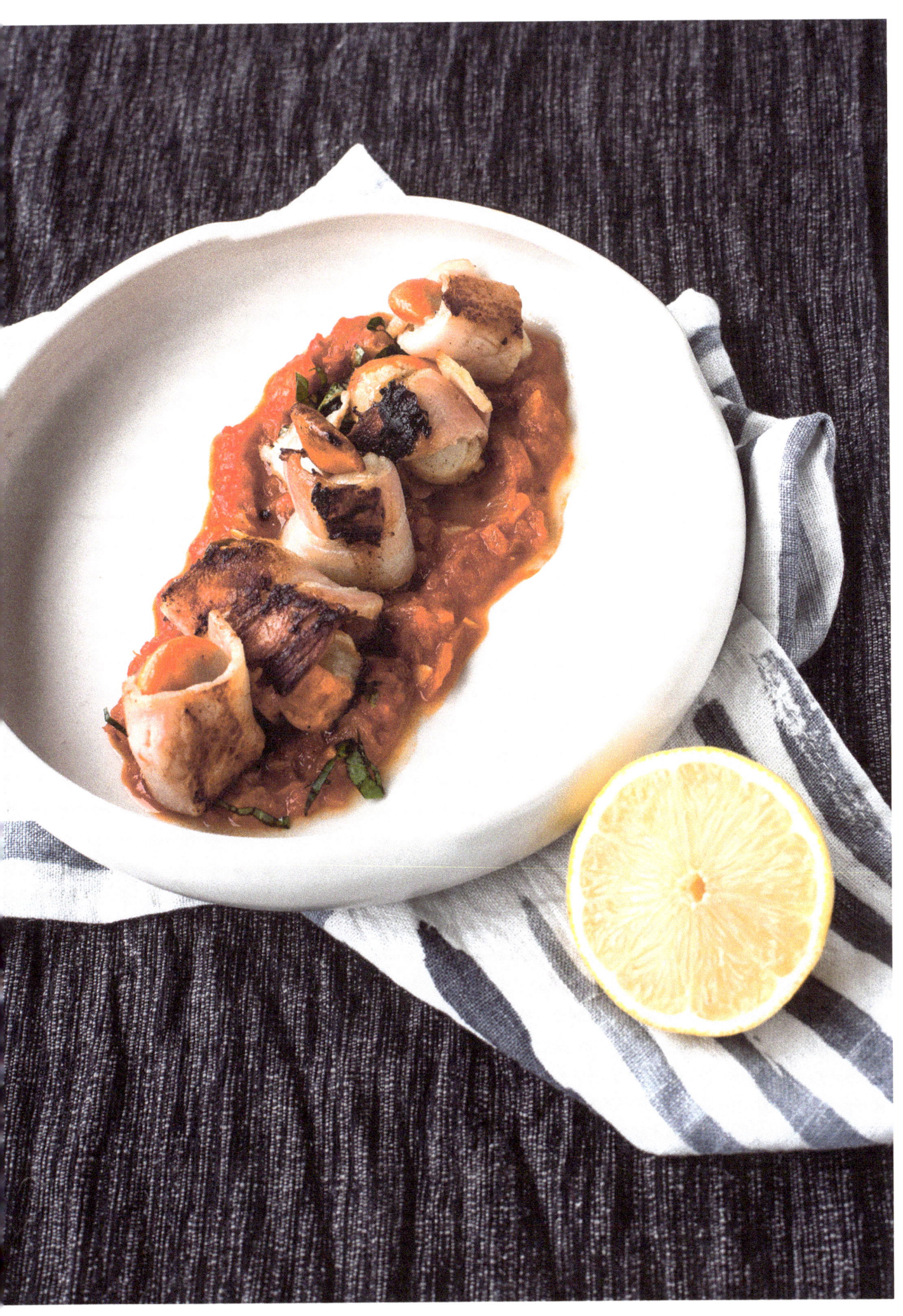

Garlic Buttered Scallops on Fillet Steak with Hollandaise

SERVES 4

This is my take on the classic 'beef and reef' dish. Cooking time for the steak will vary depending on the thickness of the fillet. The most accurate way to test the doneness of steak, if you are not confident with the pressing method, is with a meat thermometer. However, resist the temptation to poke the steak repeatedly as moisture is lost with each jab. A temperature guide is, rare – 45 to 50°C, medium – 60 to 65°C and well done – 70 to 75°C. For optimum flavour and texture, adhere to the short cooking time of the scallops and also cook them just before serving.

HOLLANDAISE

3 egg yolks

25ml white wine vinegar

150ml clarified (or melted) butter

salt and pepper

STEAK

600-800 gram beef fillet

extra virgin olive oil for pan-frying

400 grams scallops (meat only)

60 grams butter

2 cloves garlic

salt and pepper

To make the hollandaise sauce, place a heatproof bowl over a saucepan of slowly simmering water. Add the egg yolks and vinegar to the bowl, and whisk until light and fluffy, without scrambling the eggs. Melt the butter and slowly drizzle into the egg mixture whilst whisking, to create a smooth, thick sauce. Season with salt and pepper.

Allow the beef to come to room temperature before cooking. To cook the beef, cut the fillet into 4 steaks. Heat a grill, pan or the barbeque to a medium-hot heat. Brush the steaks with extra virgin olive oil. Seal the steaks on both sides for 2 minutes. Lower the heat and continue to cook, turning once or twice until they have almost reached your preferred level of doneness. Remove the steak from the heat when they are still slightly underdone, and wrap in foil to rest for 10 minutes before serving.

To cook the scallops, melt the butter in a heavy-based pan over medium heat, crush the garlic, add a good pinch of salt and pepper and sauté for 2 minutes, or until soft. Increase the heat, add the scallops and cook for 1 minute on each side.

Serve immediately with the hot steak, hollandaise and steamed greens on the side.

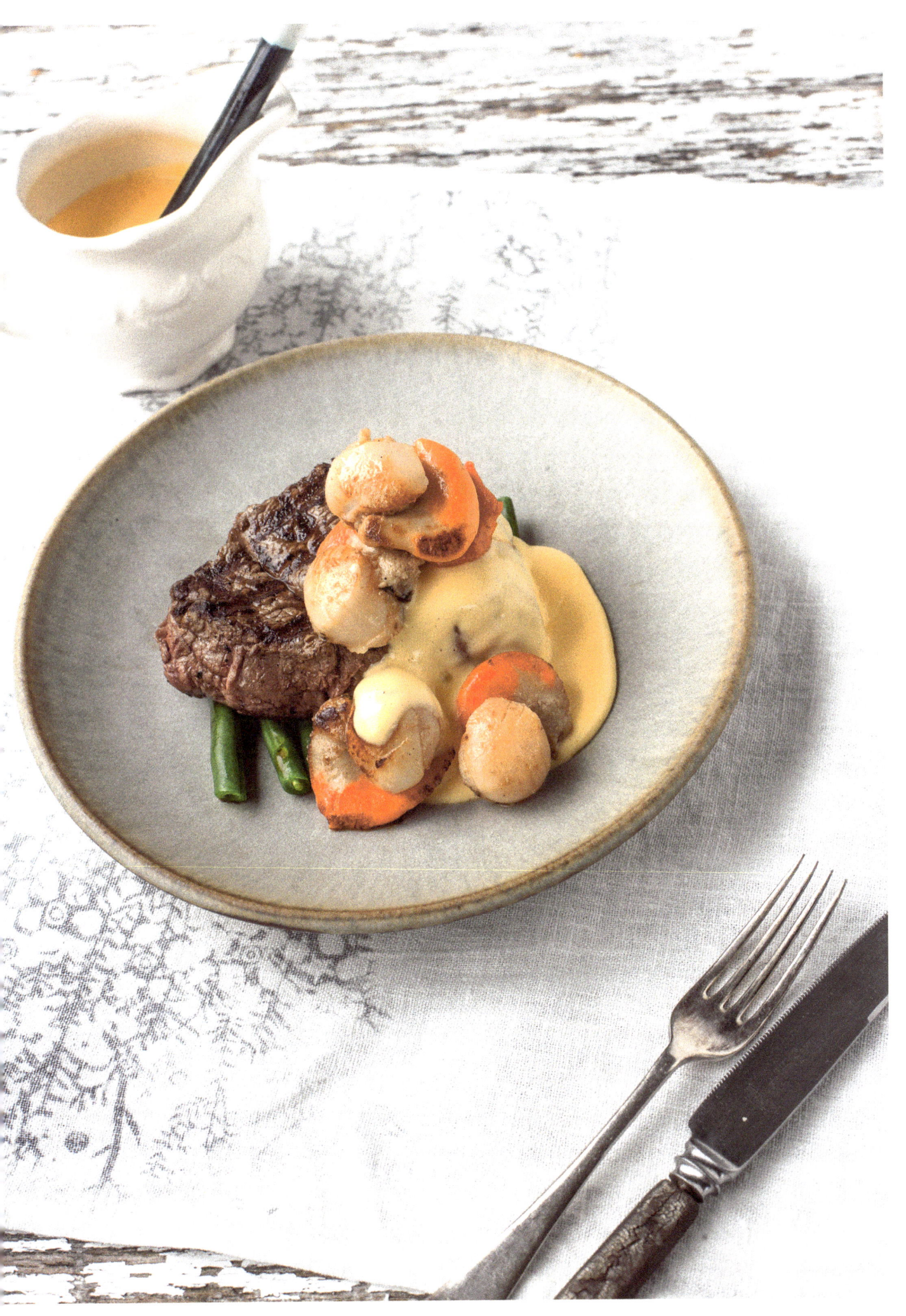

Mussels in Dill and Coconut Curry with Rice Noodles

SERVES 4

This is an extremely versatile recipe. You can substitute any seafood or chicken for the mussels, and add your favourite vegetables for a quick meal. The quantity of curry paste here makes more than you need for a single recipe, however it keeps well in the fridge and is a great standby. When making the paste, it is best to use a bunch of coriander with the roots still attached, as they add an authentic and complex flavor to the paste.

CURRY PASTE

1 small Spanish onion

6 cloves garlic

½ bunch coriander

1 bunch dill

½ bunch basil

5 birds-eye chilies

80 grams almonds

50ml extra virgin olive oil

MUSSELS AND COCONUT CURRY

2 cups cooked rice noodles

2 tablespoons extra virgin olive oil

1 onion

1 kilogram mussels

4 tablespoons curry paste

500ml seafood or vegetable stock

500ml coconut cream

2 cups chopped greens (bok choy, spinach, tat soi or silverbeet)

TO SERVE

chopped coriander

sliced red chilli

To make the curry paste, peel and roughly chop the onion and peel the garlic cloves. Remove any dirty roots from the coriander, dill and basil and roughly chop the leaves, stems and remaining roots. Add all curry paste ingredients to a food processor and blend until a smooth paste is formed. Transfer the paste to a glass jar and top with a little more extra virgin olive oil. The paste will last in the fridge for a few weeks.

Prepare the rice noodles according to packet instructions. Chop the greens, and finely slice the onion. Wash and de-beard the mussels if necessary.

To cook the dish, heat a wok over high heat. Add the extra virgin olive oil, onion and mussels, then add the curry paste and cook for a few minutes. Add the stock and coconut cream. Simmer for a few minutes or until the mussels open. Toss through the pre-cooked rice noodles and greens and serve immediately, sprinkled with additional coriander and sliced chilli.

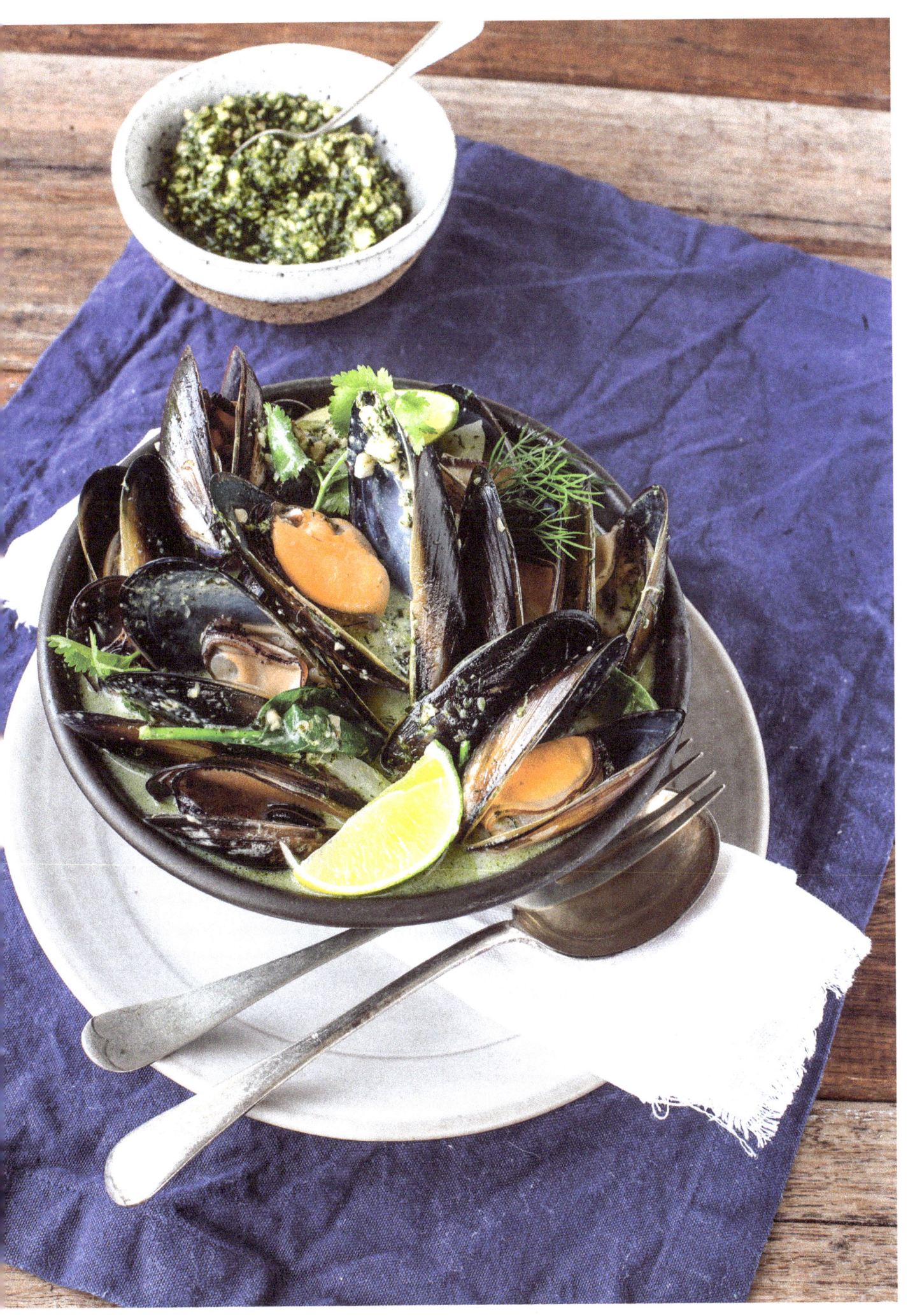

Mussels with Pumpkin Ravioli, Brown Butter and Asparagus

SERVES 4

It is really worth making the pasta by hand for this ravioli, it's silky texture is a luxurious treat.

RAVIOLI FILLING

300 grams pumpkin

1 tablespoon extra virgin olive oil

1 teaspoon basil

1 teaspoon oregano

1 clove garlic

½ cup shaved parmesan cheese

100 grams ricotta cheese

salt and pepper

RAVIOLI DOUGH

200 grams plain flour

1 tablespoon extra virgin olive oil

2 eggs

1 egg (for egg wash)

SAUCE

2 bunches fresh asparagus

2 cloves garlic

2 tablespoons sage

1 tablespoon extra virgin olive oil

1 kilogram mussels, de-bearded and scrubbed

100 grams butter

salt and pepper

½ cup additional shaved parmesan cheese

To make the ravioli filling, pre-heat the oven to 180°C. Remove the skin from the pumpkin and dice into 1 cm cubes. Pour extra virgin olive oil into a baking tray, add the pumpkin and toss lightly in the oil to coat the pieces. Bake for 25 minutes or until golden brown. Set aside to cool. Chop the basil and oregano, crush the garlic and toss with the cooled pumpkin and cheeses. Season to taste with salt and pepper.

Use a food processor to make the pasta dough. Place the flour in the food processor. Turn on the processor and with the motor running, add the extra virgin olive oil and the eggs and continue blending until the mixture comes together to form a firm dough. If the mixture seems too wet, knead in a little more flour by hand on a floured bench.

Using a pasta machine set at number 1 (or at the widest setting) feed the dough through the machine in small batches. Repeat this process 3-4 more times, increasing the setting each time until the pasta is approximately 2mm thick and silky smooth. Dust the bench with flour and carefully lay the lengths of dough aside until needed.

Crack the egg and beat in a bowl with a fork to make the egg wash. To create the ravioli, work with one sheet of pasta dough at a time. Form teaspoons of the pumpkin mixture into balls, and lay these neatly down one long side of the pasta dough, approximately 8cm apart. Brush the other side with the egg mixture and carefully fold the pasta dough over the ravioli mixture, pressing down around the mix. Use a ravioli cutter to cut into individual ravioli.

To cook the ravioli, bring a large saucepan of water to the boil and add one teaspoon of salt. Cook the ravioli for approximately 4 minutes. If you wish to cook the ravioli in advance, cook according to the directions above, cool and roll in a little extra virgin olive oil. Reheat in boiling water when ready to serve.

When you are ready to serve, cut the woody ends off the asparagus and peel the stems, crush the garlic and finely shred the sage. Heat the oil in a large, heavy based frying pan over moderate heat. Sauté the asparagus, garlic and mussels until the mussels start to open. Add the sage, butter, salt and pepper and continue to cook until all of the mussels are cooked and opened. The butter will start to brown during this process to create the sauce. If some of the mussels don't open, insert the tip of a knife and twist to open the shells.

If reheating the ravioli, return to a large saucepan of boiling water and cook for 1 minute.

Toss the mussels and asparagus mixture through the hot ravioli and serve immediately topped with the additional parmesan cheese.

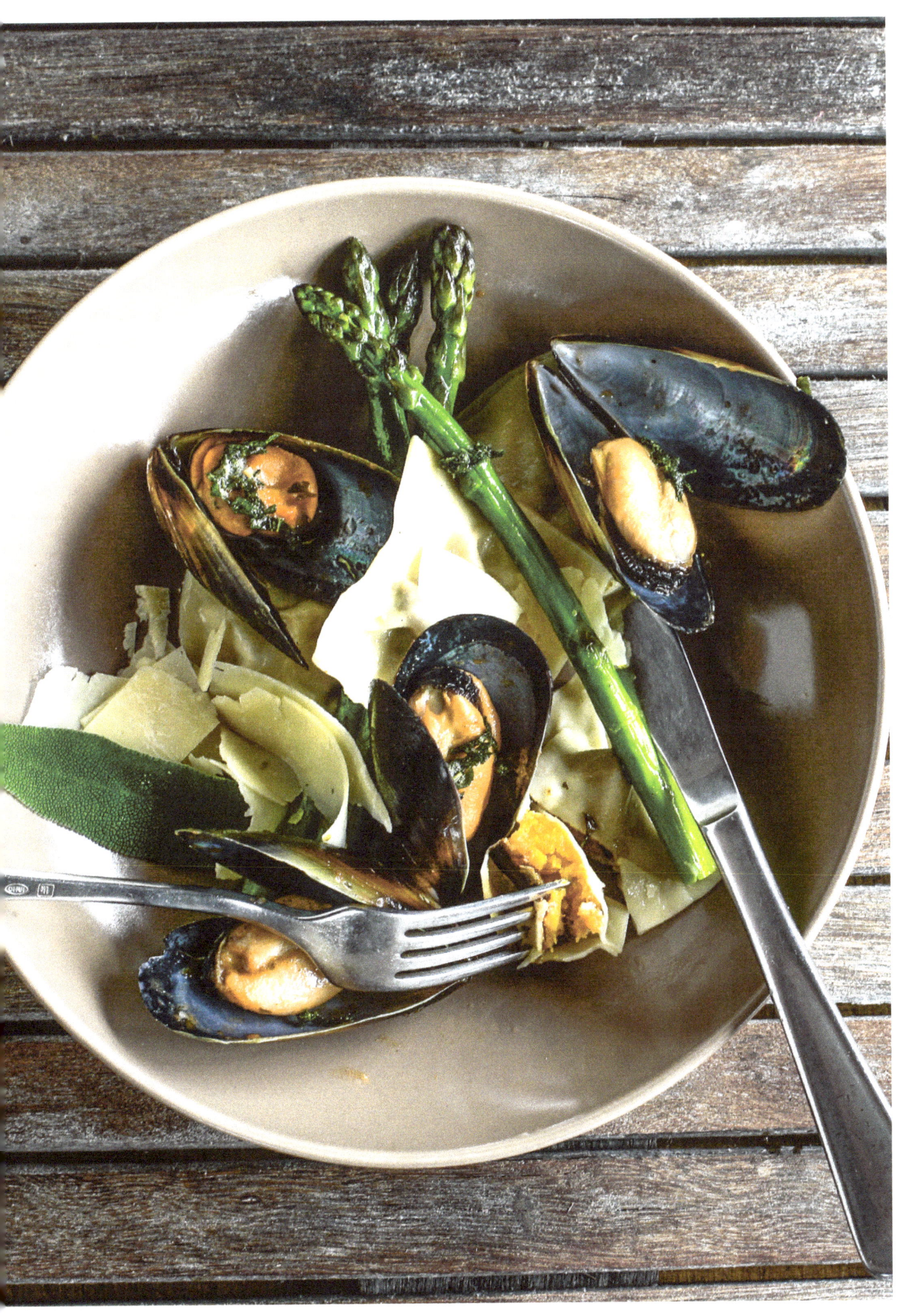

Black Lip Mussels in a White Wine, Caper, Prosciutto, Tomato, Cream Sauce with Spinach Fettuccini

SERVES 4

This recipe was the most popular dish on my menu at The Mussel Boys. It stayed on the menu the entire time I owned the restaurant, with large batches of pasta being hand rolled twice a day during the busy summer days.

PASTA

200 grams plain flour

1 tablespoon extra virgin olive oil

2 eggs

SAUCE

1 medium onion

3 cloves garlic

3 large tomatoes

3 slices prosciutto

1 tablespoon basil

1 teaspoon oregano

1 kilogram live mussels

1 tablespoon extra virgin olive oil

½ cup white wine

2 cups cream

2 tablespoons capers

cracked pepper

TO SERVE

100 grams shaved parmesan

Use a food processor to make the pasta dough. Place the flour in the food processor. Turn on the processor and with the motor running, add the extra virgin olive oil and the eggs. Continue blending until the mixture comes together to form a firm dough. If the mixture seems too wet or sticky to handle, knead in a little more flour by hand on a floured bench.

To roll the pasta, divide the dough into 4 portions. Using a pasta machine set at number 1 (or at the widest setting) feed each portion of the dough through the machine. Repeat this process with each portion of pasta on each setting, until you reach setting number 6 (or the highest setting on your machine). The pasta should be silky smooth and slightly elastic. Cut the pasta into fettuccini strips using the appropriate cutter on the pasta machine. Dust the bench with flour and carefully lay the lengths of dough aside until needed.

To cook the fettuccini, bring a large saucepan of salted water to the boil and cook the fettuccini for 4 minutes. Alternatively, the pasta can be cooked in advance, even the day before it is required. To do so, simply cook the fettuccini as above, cool and roll in a little extra virgin olive oil and refrigerate until required. Reheat the fettuccini in the sauce when you are ready to serve the dish.

To cook the sauce, peel and dice the onion, peel and crush the garlic, dice the tomato, slice the prosciutto, shred the basil and oregano and de-beard the mussels. Heat the extra virgin olive oil in a large pan over medium heat and sauté the onions, garlic and prosciutto in the extra virgin olive oil for about a minute, or until the onion is cooked. Add the tomato and mussels and cook for one minute, then add the wine, cream and capers. Cook for 3 minutes and as the mussels are starting to open add the pasta, basil and oregano and season with pepper. Take care with adding salt as the prosciutto and capers add saltiness to the dish. Cook for approximately 10 minutes, or until the sauce has reduced and thickened, the mussels are ready and the pasta is hot.

Serve immediately, topped with shaved parmesan cheese.

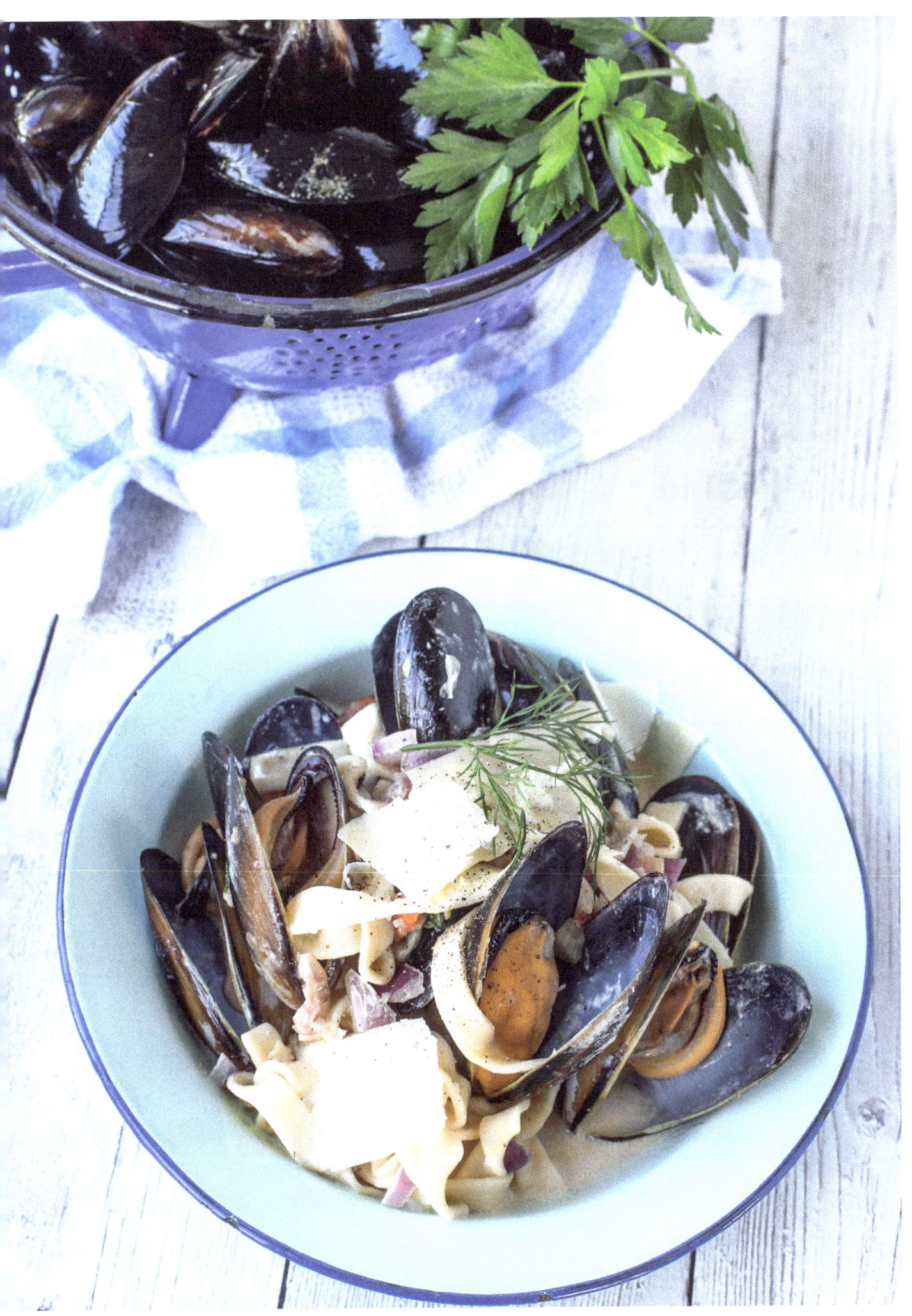

Chilli Mussels with Spaghetti, Chorizo and Tomato Sauce

SERVES 4

The tomato sauce for this dish can be made up to two days in advance, and stored in the refrigerator.

TOMATO SAUCE

½ onion

3 large garlic cloves

3 birds eye chilies

1 tablespoon basil

1 tablespoon oregano

25ml extra virgin olive oil

400 grams crushed tomatoes

SPAGHETTI

200 grams plain flour

1 tablespoon extra virgin olive oil

2 eggs

CHILLI MUSSELS

1 kilogram mussels, de-bearded and scrubbed

1 spicy chorizo sausage

25ml extra virgin olive oil

100ml white wine

salt and pepper

½ cup shaved parmesan

To make the tomato sauce, chop the onion, crush the garlic, and finely chop the chilies and herbs. Heat the extra virgin olive oil in a saucepan over low heat, and sweat the onion, garlic, and chilies until soft. Add the tomato and herbs, and simmer gently for 15 minutes.

Use a food processor to make the pasta dough. Place the flour in the food processor. Turn on the processor and with the motor running, add the extra virgin olive oil and the eggs. Continue blending until the mixture comes together to form a firm dough. If the mixture seems too wet or sticky to handle, knead in a little more flour by hand on a floured bench.

To roll the pasta, divide the dough into 4 portions. Using a pasta machine set at number 1 (or at the widest setting) feed each portion of the dough through the machine. Repeat this process with each portion of pasta on each setting, until you reach setting number 6, (or the highest setting on your machine) the pasta should be silky smooth and slightly elastic. Cut the pasta into spaghetti strips using the appropriate cutter on the pasta machine. Dust the bench with flour and carefully lay the lengths of dough aside until needed.

To cook the spaghetti, bring a large saucepan of salted water to the boil and cook the spaghetti for 4 minutes. Alternatively the pasta can be cooked in advance, even the day before it is required. To do so, simply cook the spaghetti as above, cool and roll in a little extra virgin olive oil and refrigerate until required. Reheat the spaghetti in the sauce when you are ready to serve the dish.

To finish, de-beard the mussels and finely dice the chorizo. Heat the oil in a large, heavy-based pan over medium heat, and add the mussels, chorizo and white wine. When the mussels have started to open, add the tomato sauce. Toss through the pasta and top with parmesan to serve.

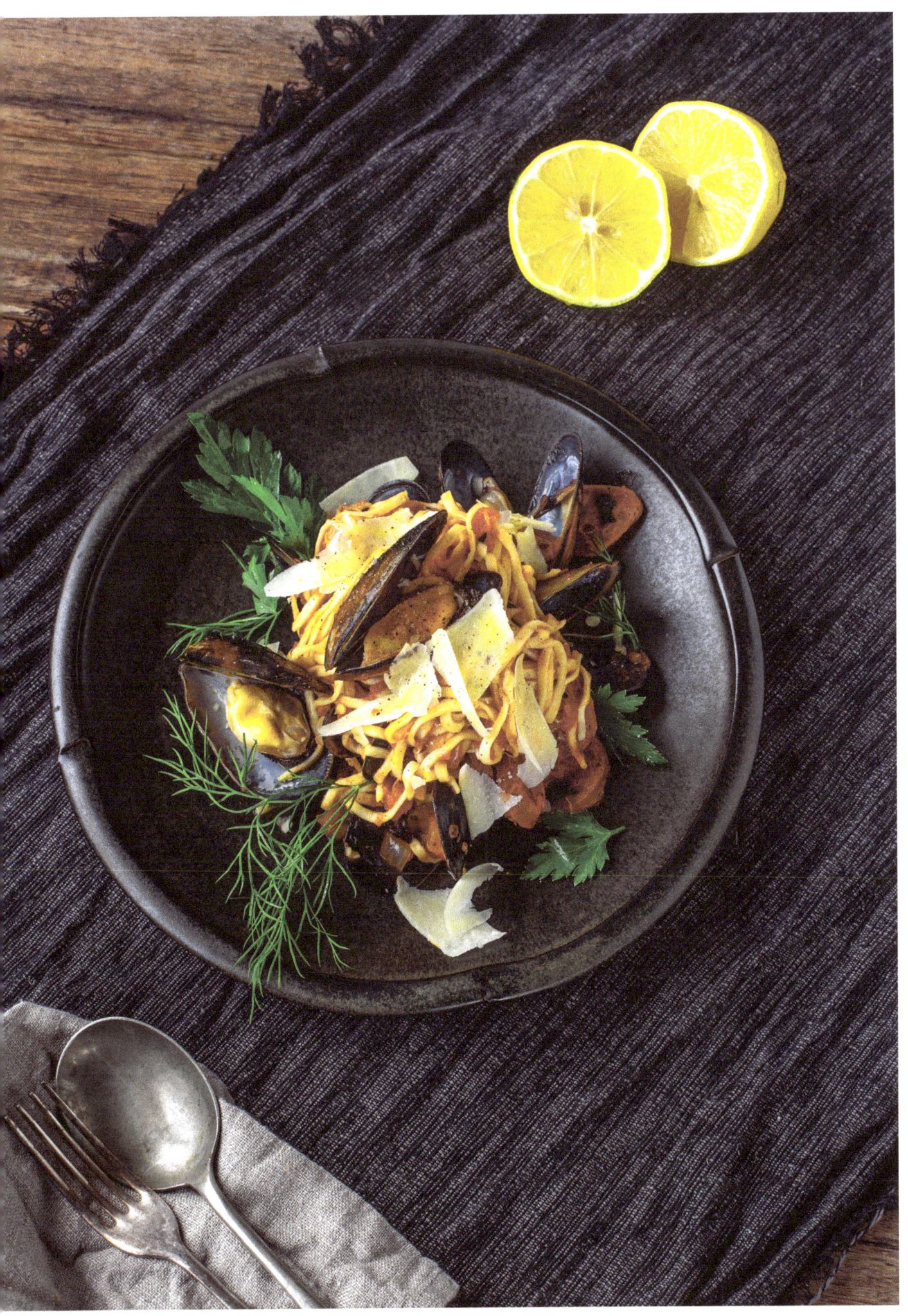

Panko Crumbed Abalone

SERVES 4 AS AN ENTRÉE OR LIGHT MEAL

This very simple and delicious method of cooking abalone is also quite adaptable. Try adding different dry spice mixes such as harissa or Japanese 7 spice to the flour. My personal favourite method is to stuff it with garlic butter before crumbing and cook it on the barbeque. Perfect summer yumminess!

2-3 abalone

1 egg

200ml milk

300 grams panko bread crumbs

salt and pepper

200 grams plain flour

extra virgin olive oil for shallow frying

TO SERVE

Asian style salad, see page 80

To tenderise the abalone, fold a tea towel in half and lay on the bench. Cut the lip off the abalone and place it in between the halves of the tea towel. Give the abalone 4-5 good hits with a meat mallet on each side. The abalone should now feel considerably softer, as the muscle tissue will have been broken.

Make an egg wash by whisking together the egg and milk. Season the panko crumbs well with a good pinch of salt and pepper.

To crumb the abalone, dip each fish in the flour and shake off any excess. Next, dip the abalone into the egg wash and again shake off any excess. Finally, dip the abalone into the breadcrumbs, ensuring the whole fish is well coated. Repeat this for each abalone.

To cook the abalone, heat a dash of oil in a heavy-based frying pan, or on the flat grill of a barbeque, over medium heat. Fry the abalone for 1-2 minutes on each side, or until cooked through. The meat should be white when sliced.

Cut into thin slices and serve with Asian salad.

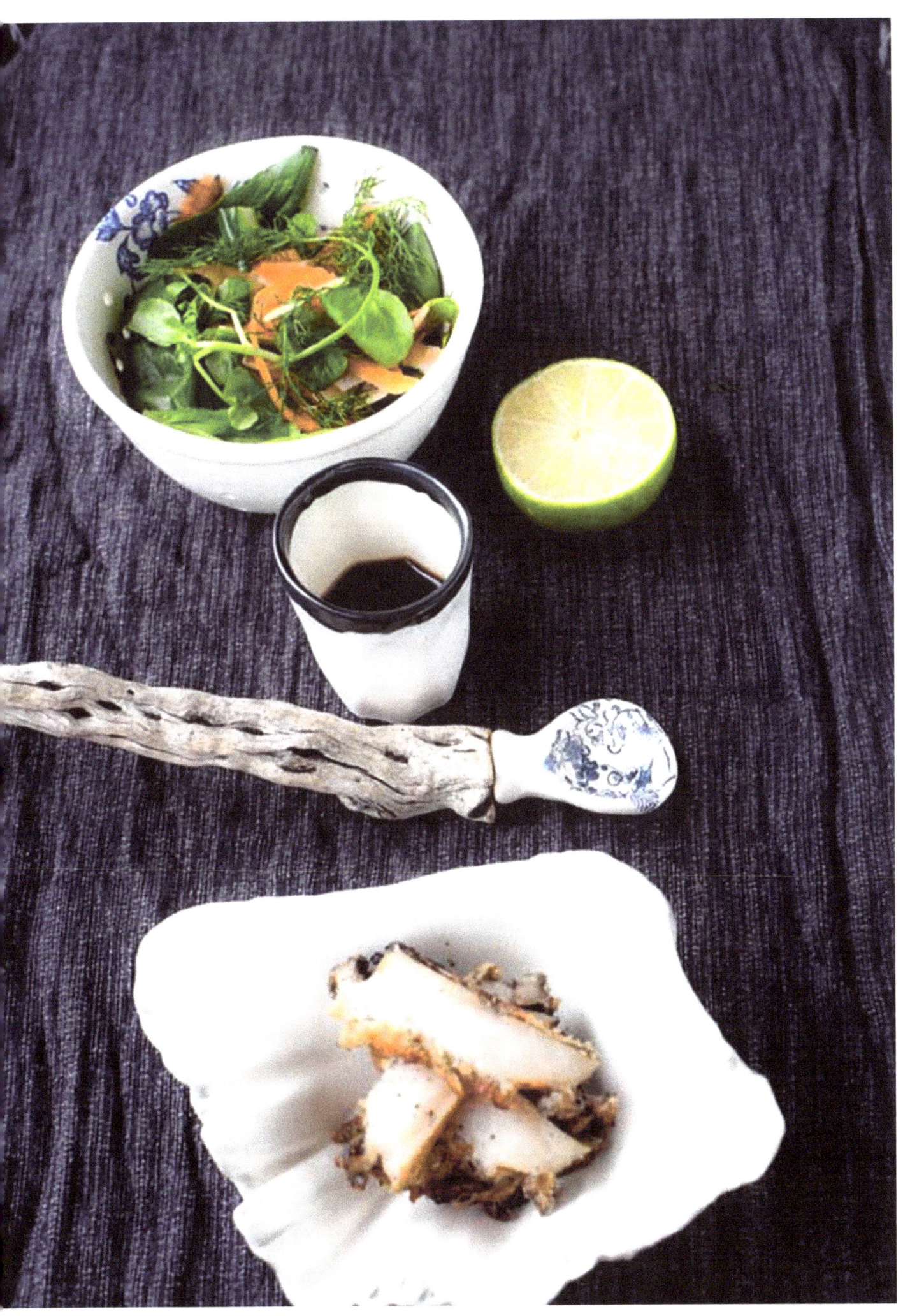

Abalone with a Lime, Watercress and Goats Cheese Salad

SERVES 4 AS AN ENTRÉE OR LIGHT MEAL

For best results, cook the abalone just before serving this salad.

3-4 abalone

extra virgin olive oil for cooking

SALAD

80 grams of chevre, or goats cheese

1 large cucumber

100 grams watercress

DRESSING

juice of 1 lime

1 tablespoon white wine vinegar

2 tablespoons light extra virgin olive oil

salt and pepper

To prepare the salad, finely slice the cucumber, and wash and dry the watercress. Crumble or dice the chevre. Arrange the cucumber, watercress and goats cheese on plate. To make the dressing, combine all dressing ingredients and mix well.

To prepare and cook the abalone, cut the lip off the abalone. Thinly slice the whole abalone, cutting across the fish. Using a meat mallet, bash each slice on each side.

Close to serving time, heat the extra virgin olive oil in a pan over a medium-hot heat. Season the abalone slices with salt and pepper and flash fry, for 30 seconds on each side, until golden brown and cooked.

Serve the abalone immediately on the prepared salad and top with dressing.

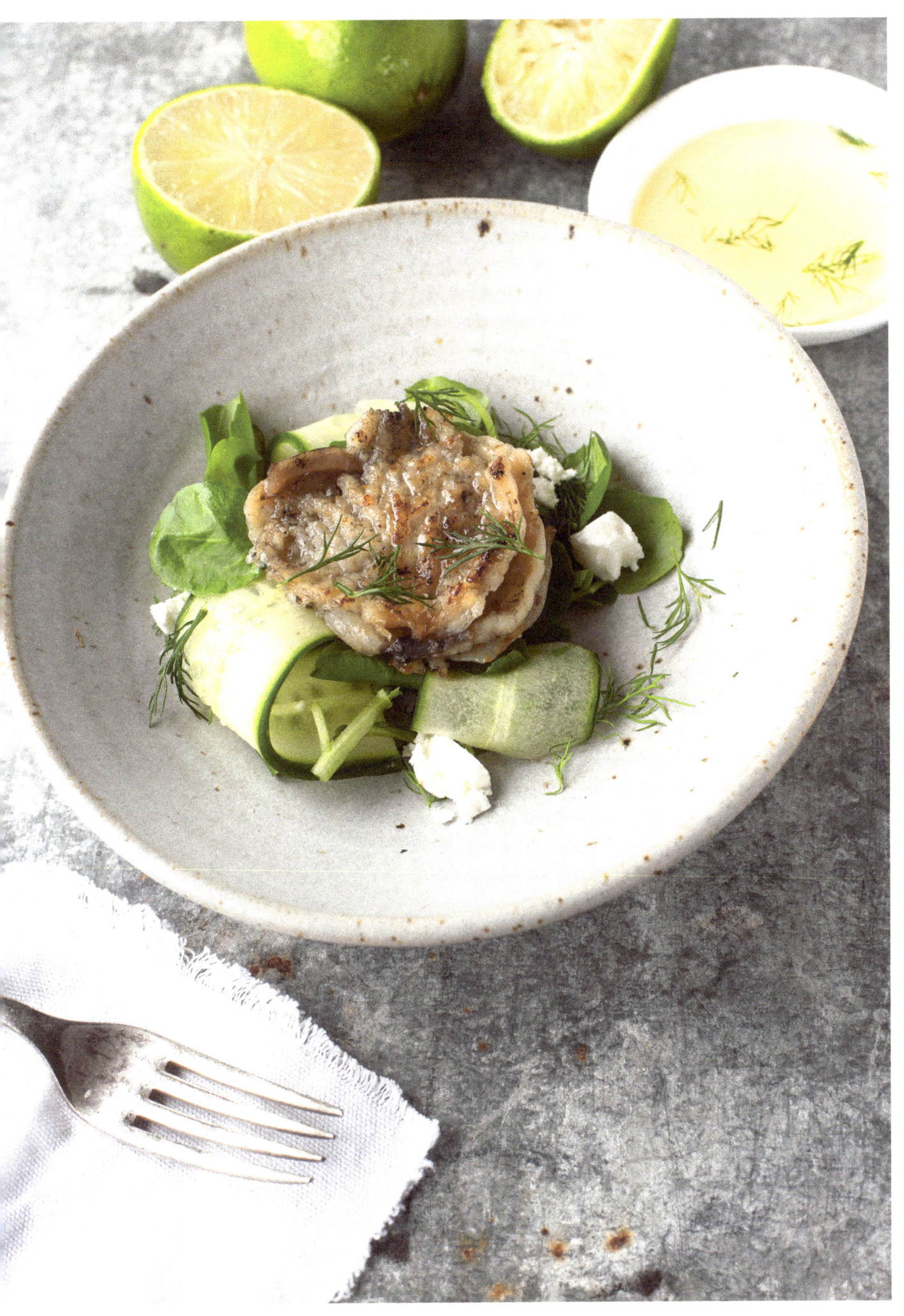

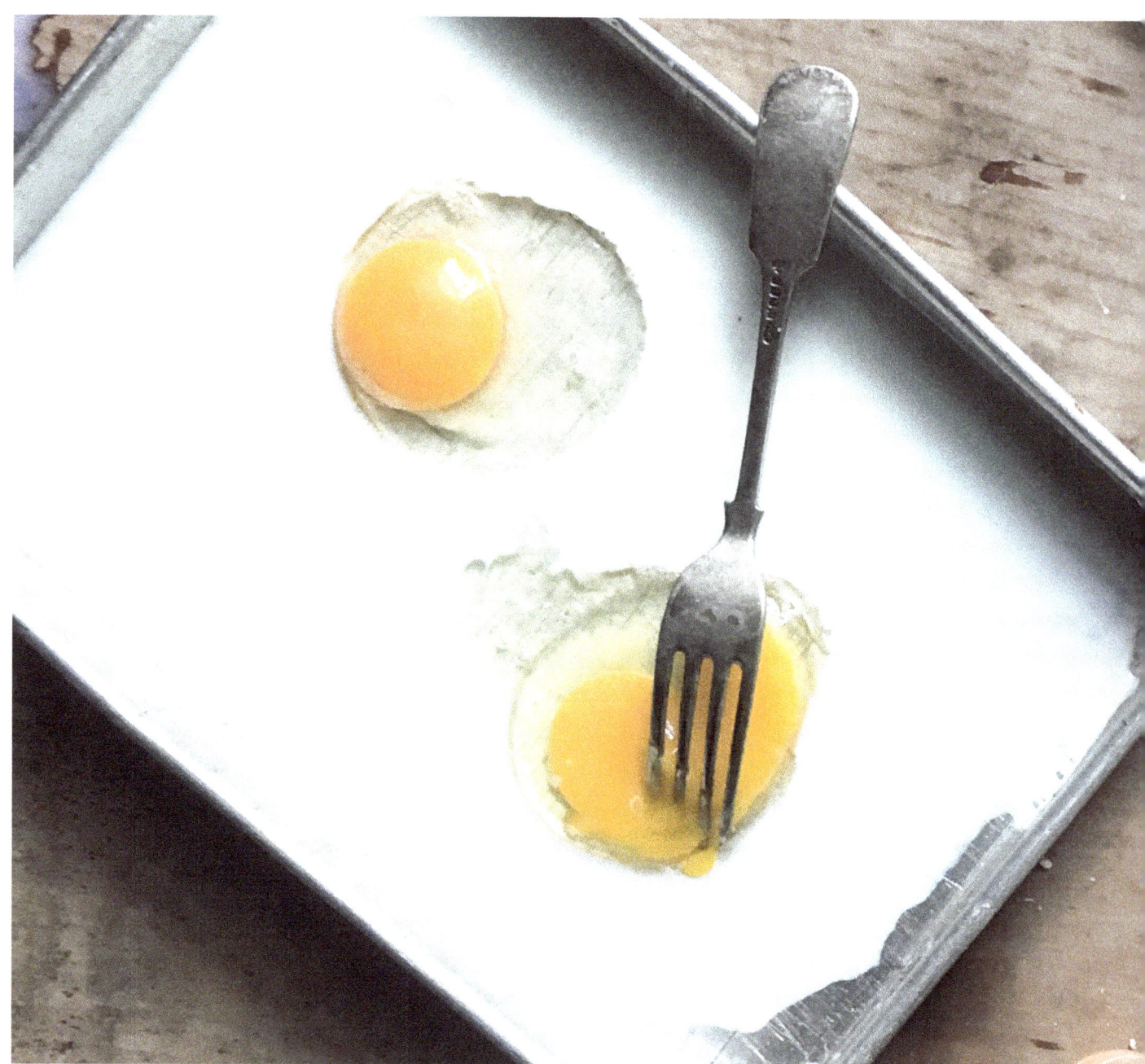

Pantry Staples

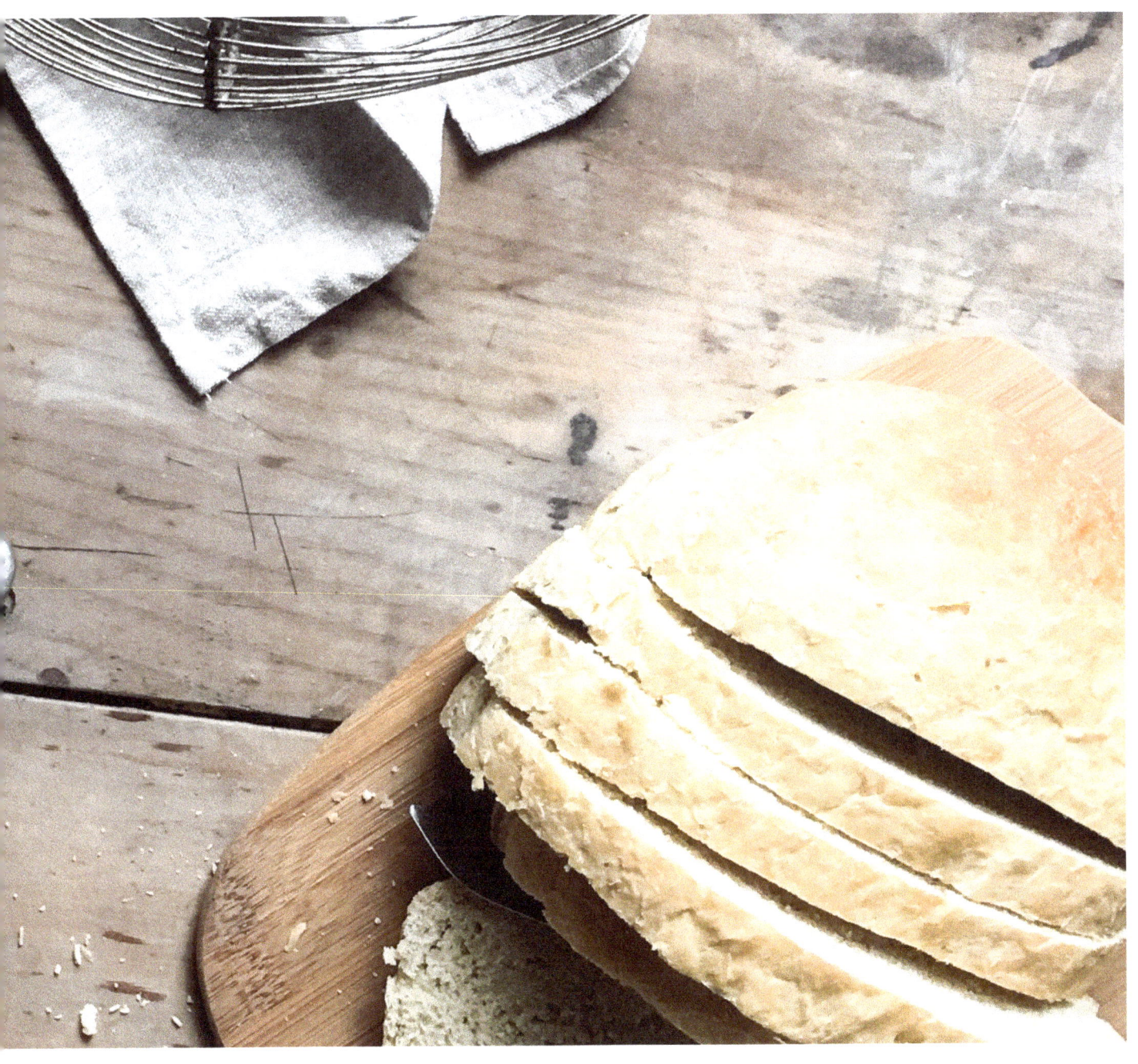

Salmon Omelette

SERVES 2-3

This lovely light recipe is perfect for lunch, or served with some fresh bread and salad it can also be a superb, fast dinner. When not in season, the fresh asparagus can be substituted with chopped spinach or silverbeet leaves. Fresh or smoked salmon can also be used here.

6 large eggs

100ml cream

1 tablespoon fresh tarragon

salt and pepper

12 spears fresh asparagus

1 clove garlic

½ medium brown onion

1 teaspoon butter

150 grams mozzarella cheese

200 grams canned salmon

Whisk eggs and cream in a bowl until combined. Add the finely chopped tarragon and a pinch of salt and pepper, and whisk to combine.

Cut the woody ends off the asparagus spears, crush the garlic and finely slice the onion.

Using a heavy based, medium sized frying pan, melt the butter over moderate heat and sauté the onion until tender.

Add the garlic and asparagus and sauté for a further 1-2 minutes or until softened. Pour the egg mixture into the pan, and top with the grated mozzarella cheese and salmon.

Cover the frying pan with a lid and cook over low heat for about 5 minutes or until cooked through.

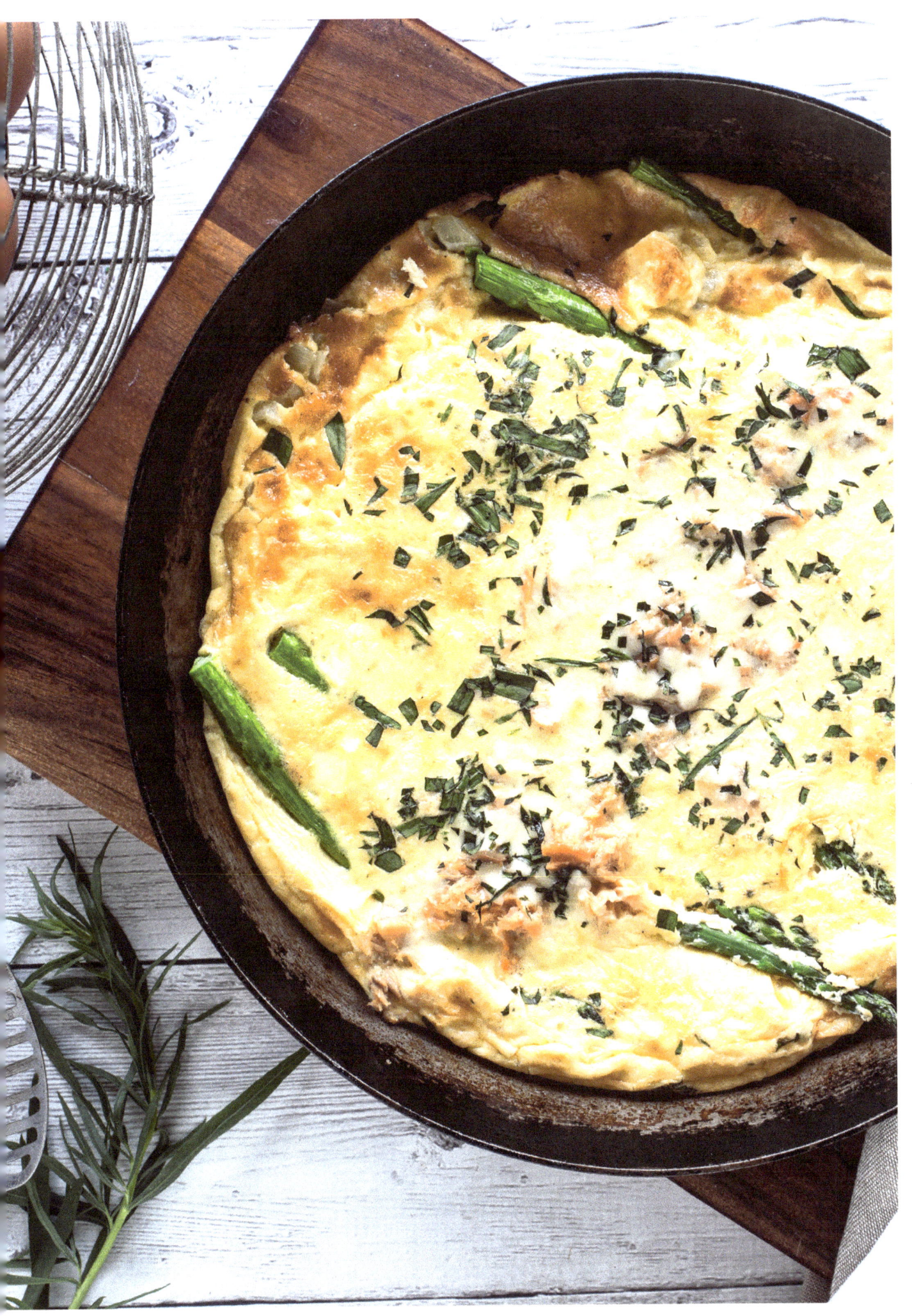

Smoked Salmon Pizza with Capers, Red Onion and Sour Cream

SERVES 4

The recipe for this pizza dough is suitable for a domestic bread maker, otherwise it can be mixed and kneaded by hand. This quantity will also make one loaf or 12 dinner rolls and can be used to make a batch of grissini. You can use white, wholemeal flour, or a mixture of both, in this recipe.

PIZZA DOUGH

3 ½ cups plain flour

1 teaspoon salt

½ teaspoon sugar

1 teaspoon dry yeast

1 teaspoon bread improver

1 tablespoon semolina

20ml milk

20ml extra virgin olive oil

320ml lukewarm water

PIZZA TOPPING

1 Spanish onion

300 grams bocconcini or mozzarella

200ml tomato passata

600 grams smoked salmon

2 tablespoons baby capers

100ml sour cream

If you are using a bread maker to make the pizza dough, place all of the dough ingredients into the breadmaker and use the basic dough setting. It will take approximately 2 hours to knead and rise. To make the dough by hand, mix the dry ingredients together and then add wet ingredients to form a rough dough. Knead for 20 minutes, or until a smooth, elastic dough is formed.

Cover with plastic wrap and leave to rise in a warm place for around one hour, or until the dough has doubled in size. Knock back and knead for 2 minutes until the dough feels tight again. Divide into portions for your pizzas – it will make 2 large pizzas or around 12 mini pizzas.

To make the pizzas, pre-heat the oven to 200°C. Finely chop the onion and grate the mozarella if necessary. Roll out each portion of dough and lay on a lightly oiled tray and top with passata, onion and cheese.

Leave to rise for a few minutes (or longer if you prefer a thicker pizza base), place on a baking tray and cook for 15-20 minutes until golden brown.

Cut into slices while still hot and top each slice with smoked salmon, capers and a dollop of sour cream.

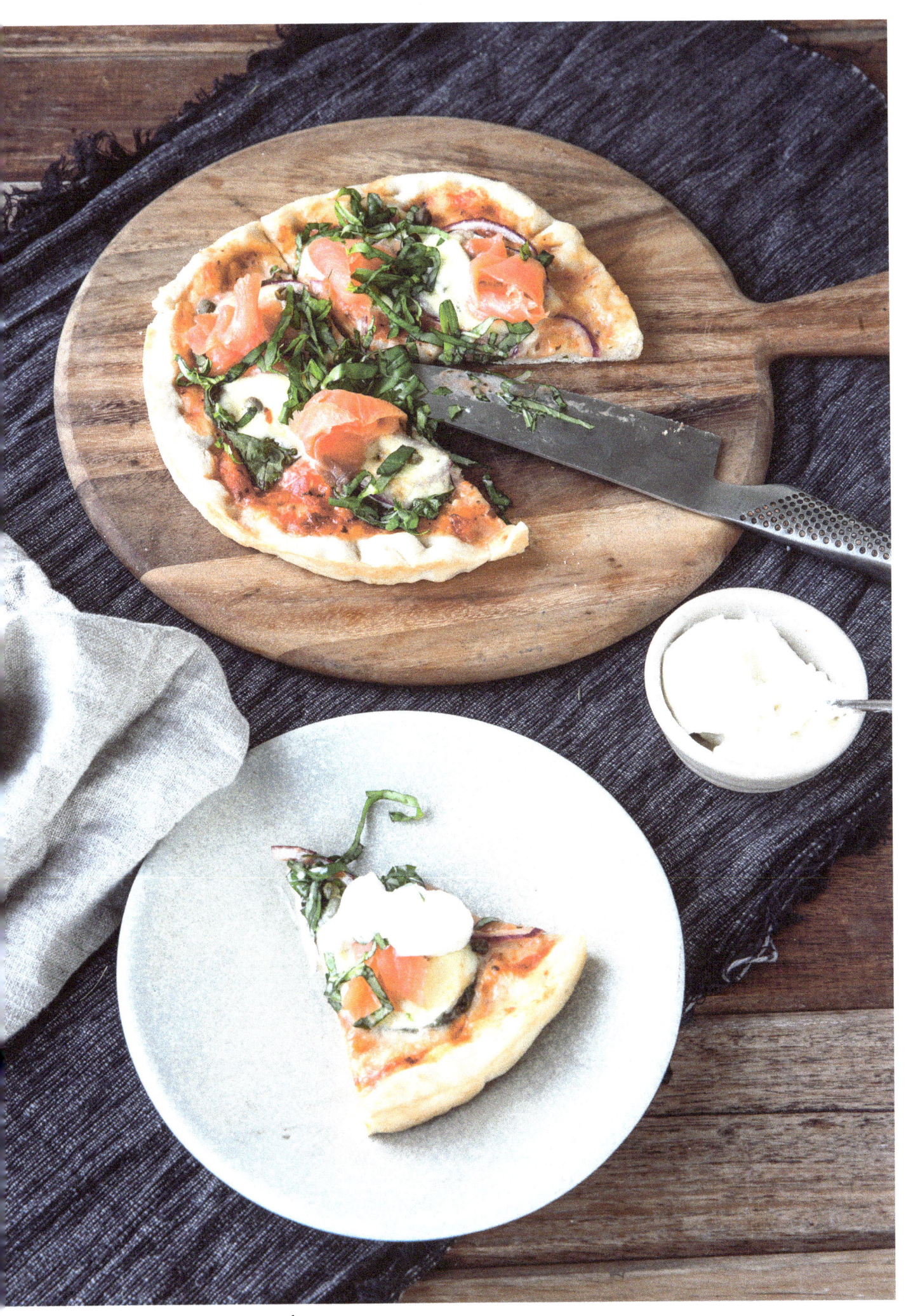

Gnocchi in Cream Sauce with Salmon

SERVES 4

This easy way of making gnocchi by boiling the potatoes is different from the traditional method, and I find it a lot easier! If you are using good quality potatoes it works brilliantly and you'll find yourself making this gnocchi all the time. To save time, you can cook the gnocchi in advance and then reheat them in boiling water when it comes time to serve.

GNOCCHI

500 grams floury potatoes, such as Kennebec

2 eggs

½ teaspoon nutmeg

1 cup plain flour

salt and pepper

SALMON SAUCE

1 tablespoon extra virgin olive oil

3 cloves garlic

1 medium brown onion

100 grams mushrooms

100ml white wine

300ml cream

50 grams sundried tomatoes

2 tablespoons basil

1 tablespoon oregano

300 grams salmon

salt and pepper

TO SERVE

100 grams parmesan cheese

To make the gnocchi, peel and dice the potatoes into 2cm cubes. Place potatoes in a saucepan, cover with water, bring to the boil and simmer for 18 minutes or until the potatoes are cooked through. Drain well and set aside to cool for a few minutes.

While the potatoes are still warm, mash well and stir through the eggs, nutmeg, flour and a pinch of salt and pepper. If the dough is too sticky to handle, add a little more flour. Using lightly floured hands, roll the dough into balls around the size of a ten cent piece, set aside on a lightly floured plate until ready to cook.

To cook the gnocchi, bring a large pot of salted water to the boil. Carefully place the gnocchi into the water and bring back to a simmer. Continue to simmer for about 4 minutes, or until cooked through, drain and set aside until ready to use.

To make the sauce, heat the extra virgin olive oil in a heavy based pan over medium heat and sauté the crushed garlic and sliced onion until tender. Add the sliced mushrooms to the pan and continue sautéing until just cooked through. Add the wine, cream and chopped sundried tomatoes and cook for about 4 minutes or until the cream starts to reduce. Add the herbs and salmon and season with salt and pepper.

To serve, toss the hot gnocchi through the sauce and serve immediately topped with grated or shaved parmesan cheese.

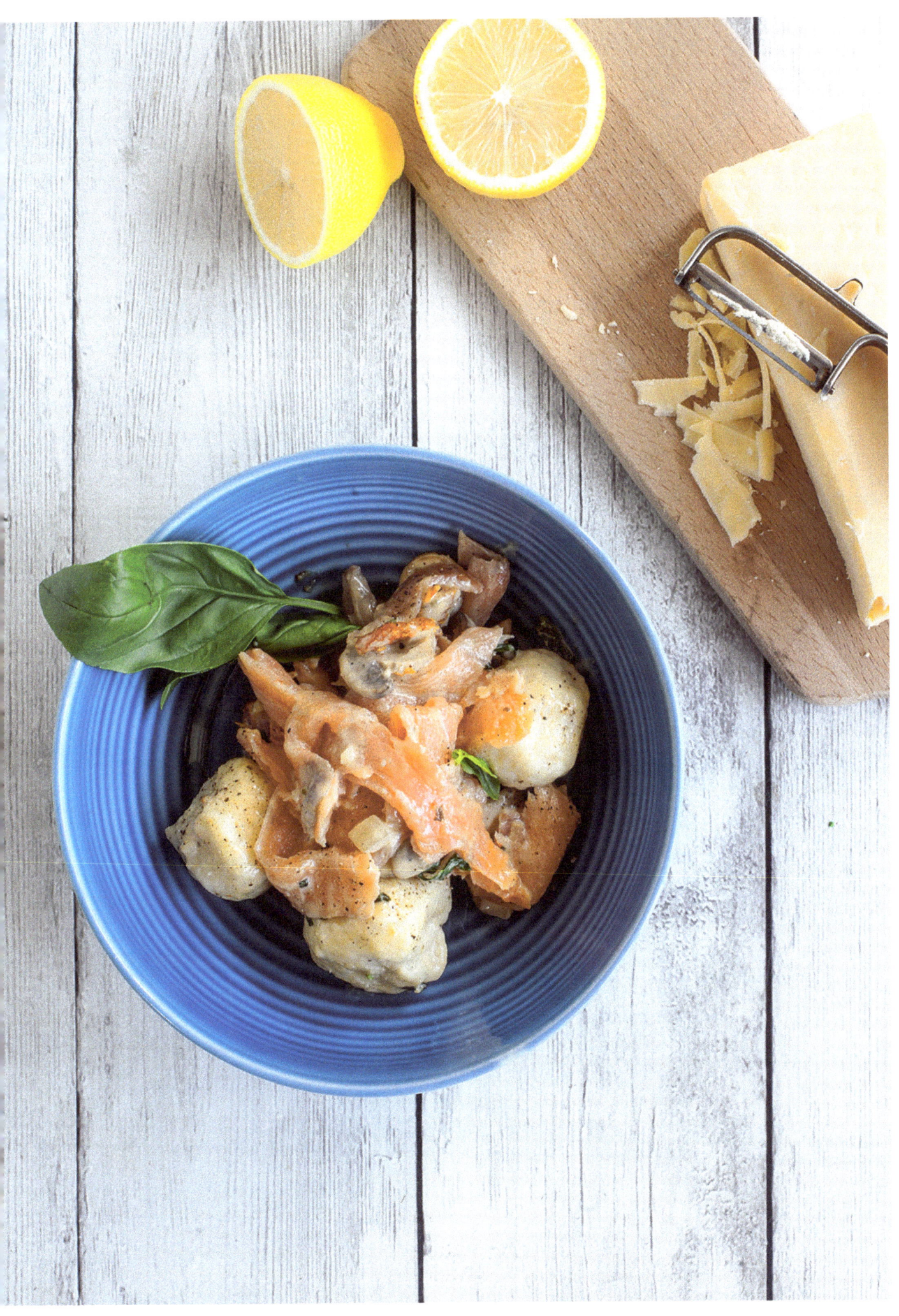

Pink Eye Potato and Salmon Salad

SERVES 4-6

This is such a versatile salad. Dress it up for a dinner party by serving it with a freshly baked salmon steak or sliced smoked salmon, or dress it down for an easy lunch by using a can of tinned salmon. Pink Eye potatoes are a highly sought after waxy variety grown in Tasmania and we always get very excited when the first Pink Eyes of the season arrive! Substitute other waxy varieties such as Bintje or Dutch Cream.

8 medium pink-eye potatoes

4 eggs

3 tablespoons sour cream

3 tablespoons mayonnaise

1 tablespoon capers

2 tablespoons dill

1 tablespoon chives

1 small red onion

salt and pepper

400 grams smoked salmon

Scrub the potatoes but do not peel. Place the whole potatoes in a saucepan, cover with water, bring to the boil and simmer for 15 minutes, or until the potatoes are cooked but still firm. Drain and cool, then cut into 1cm dice.

Hard boil the eggs by cooking in a pot of boiling water for 10 minutes. Cool the eggs and peel. Cut into quarters.

In a large bowl, mix together the sour cream and mayonnaise. Add the capers, chopped herbs, sliced onion, potatoes and egg. Stir gently to combine.

To serve, transfer the potato mixture to a serving dish. Season with salt and pepper and serve with the smoked salmon.

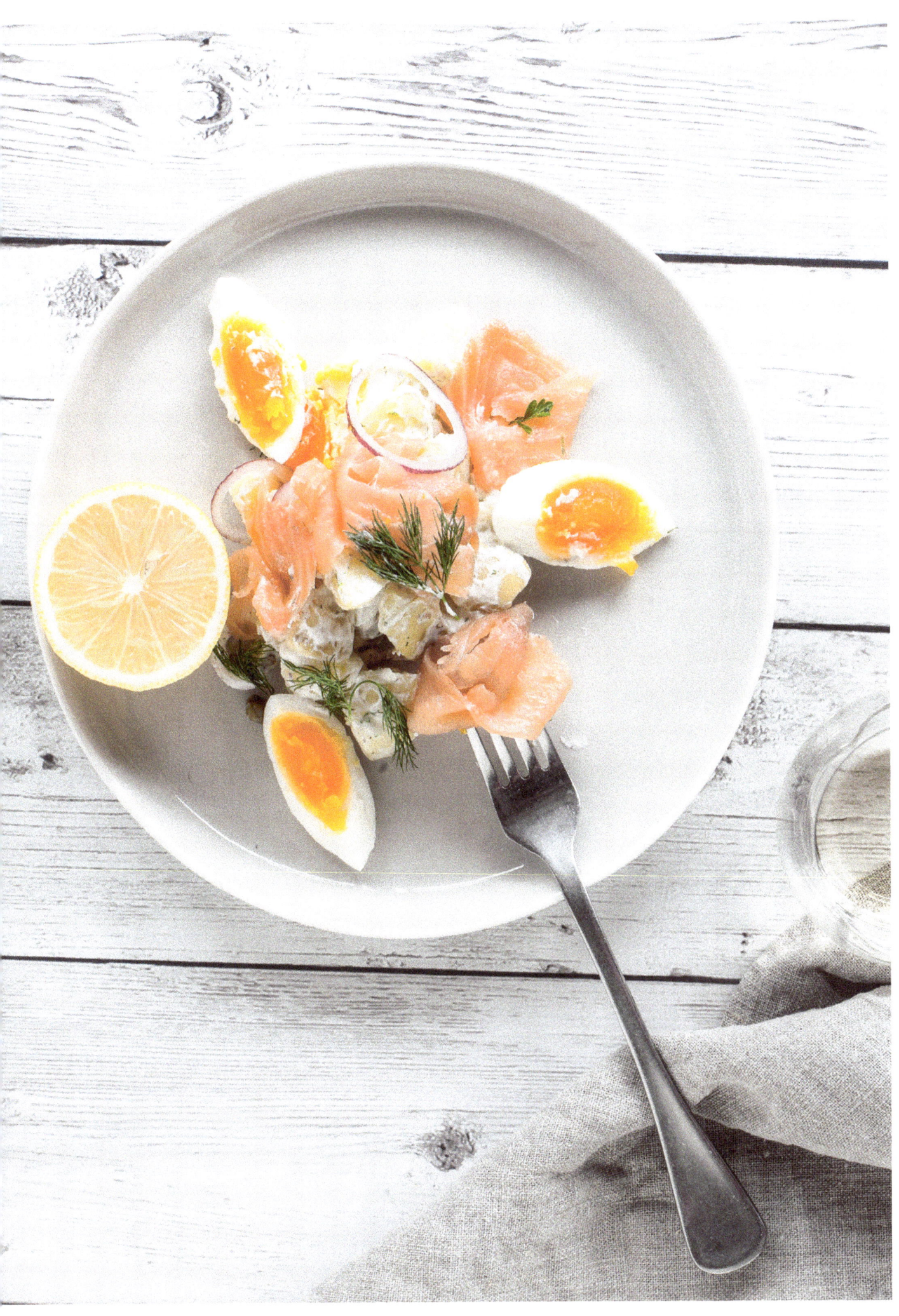

Tuna Nori Rolls

MAKES 8 LARGE ROLLS

If you haven't made sushi before, you'll find these nori rolls surprisingly easy to make. I don't use any fancy equipment or rolling mats, but simply place the rice and filling directly onto the seaweed sheets and roll with my hands. These are great in lunchboxes and a fabulous alternative to a sandwich. Try making them in advance for a super quick dinner on busy weekday evening.

SUSHI RICE

1 cup sushi rice

1 tablespoon rice wine vinegar

1 teaspoon caster sugar

4 nori sheets

FILLING

Japanese mayonnaise (such as Kewpie brand)

carrot, grated raw or cooked in strips

cucumber, sliced

spring onions, sliced

bean sprouts

avocado, sliced

salmon smoked, fresh or tinned

tuna, fresh or tinned

hard boiled eggs, in quarters

tofu, sliced

capsicum, sliced

TO SERVE

wasabi

soy sauce

pickled ginger

Sushi rice, rice wine vinegar, nori sheets, Japanese mayonnaise and tofu are generally available at supermarkets, otherwise try your local Asian grocer.

To make the sushi rice, place the rice in a colander and rinse under cold running water to wash off any excess starch. Put the rice into a heavy based saucepan with 1½ cups water. Bring to a gentle boil, reduce the heat and cook covered for about 12 minutes, or until all of the water has been absorbed. Remove from the heat and rest covered, for 10 minutes to finish cooking. Add the vinegar and sugar to the rice and fold through. To cool the rice, cover a board or tray with baking paper and spread over the rice in a thin layer.

To assemble the nori rolls, cover ⅔ of a nori sheet with a thin layer of rice. Place your filling ingredients down the middle of the rice. Add a squeeze of mayonnaise. Carefully roll the nori sheet as tightly as possible to enclose the fillings and to make a firm roll. Place into a container with the join side down, and refrigerate for 20 minutes before eating.

To serve, slice the sushi into rolls and offer wasabi, soy sauce and pickled ginger.

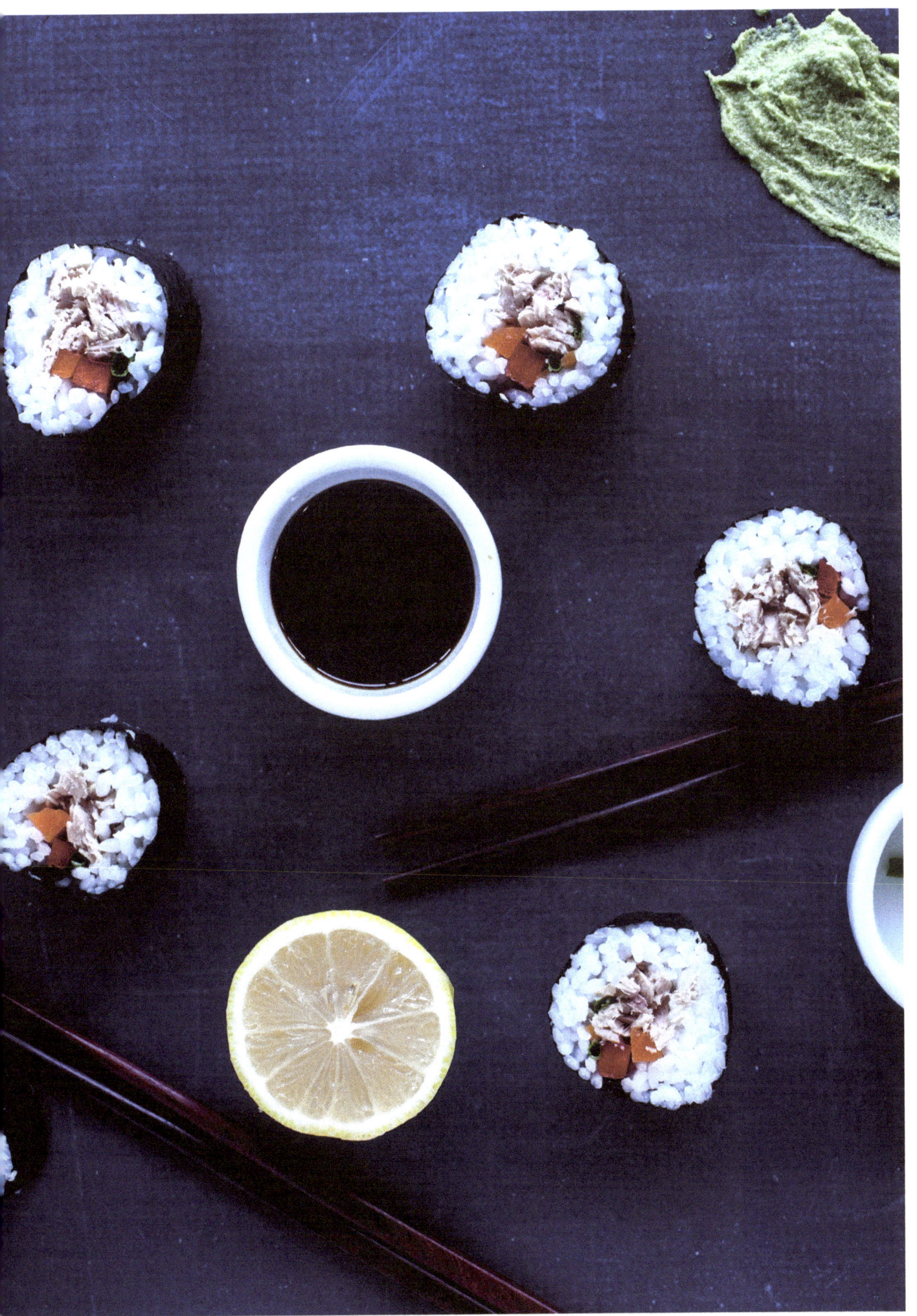

Salmon and White Bean Salad

SERVES 4

For a quick and easy dinner, use a tin of canned beans and roast red peppers from a jar. If you have more time, soak the beans the night before and roast the capsicum yourself. Unlike a salad made with salad leaves that would wilt if dressed too early, this dish would benefit from marinating overnight. This salad can be made the night before a busy day, and the salmon added right before serving.

4 x 180-200 gram salmon steaks, or 600 grams smoked or tinned salmon

SALAD

extra virgin olive oil

1 large red capsicum

2 large zucchini

1 tablespoon oregano

1 tablespoon parsley

1 tablespoon basil

2 cloves garlic

juice and zest of 1 lemon

400 grams cooked cannellini beans

100 grams feta cheese

salt and pepper

Pre-heat the oven to 180°C.

To make the salad, rub the capsicum with a small amount of extra virgin olive oil and roast in the oven for 10 minutes - or until the capsicum has softened and the skin is blackened. Remove capsicum from the oven, place in a bowl and cover with plastic wrap, this will make the capsicums easier to peel.

Once the capsicum has cooled enough to handle, peel off the skin. Remove and discard the seeds. Slice the capsicum into 5mm dice. Slice the zucchinis into a 5mm rounds and grill under a medium grill, or pan-fry in oil over medium heat, for 5 minutes, or until golden and soft.

Chop the herbs, crush the garlic and mix with the lemon juice and zest, beans, zucchini, crumbled feta and capsicum. Season with a pinch of sea salt and cracked pepper.

To cook the salmon steaks, season each steak with salt and pepper. Heat a dash of extra virgin olive oil in an oven-proof frying pan over medium-hot heat. Place the salmon skin side down in the pan and cook for a few minutes, or until the skin is crisp.

Put the frying pan into the oven for 8 minutes, or until the salmon is cooked to your liking – you may need to adjust the cooking time depending on your steaks. To serve, sit the salmon on top of the salad.

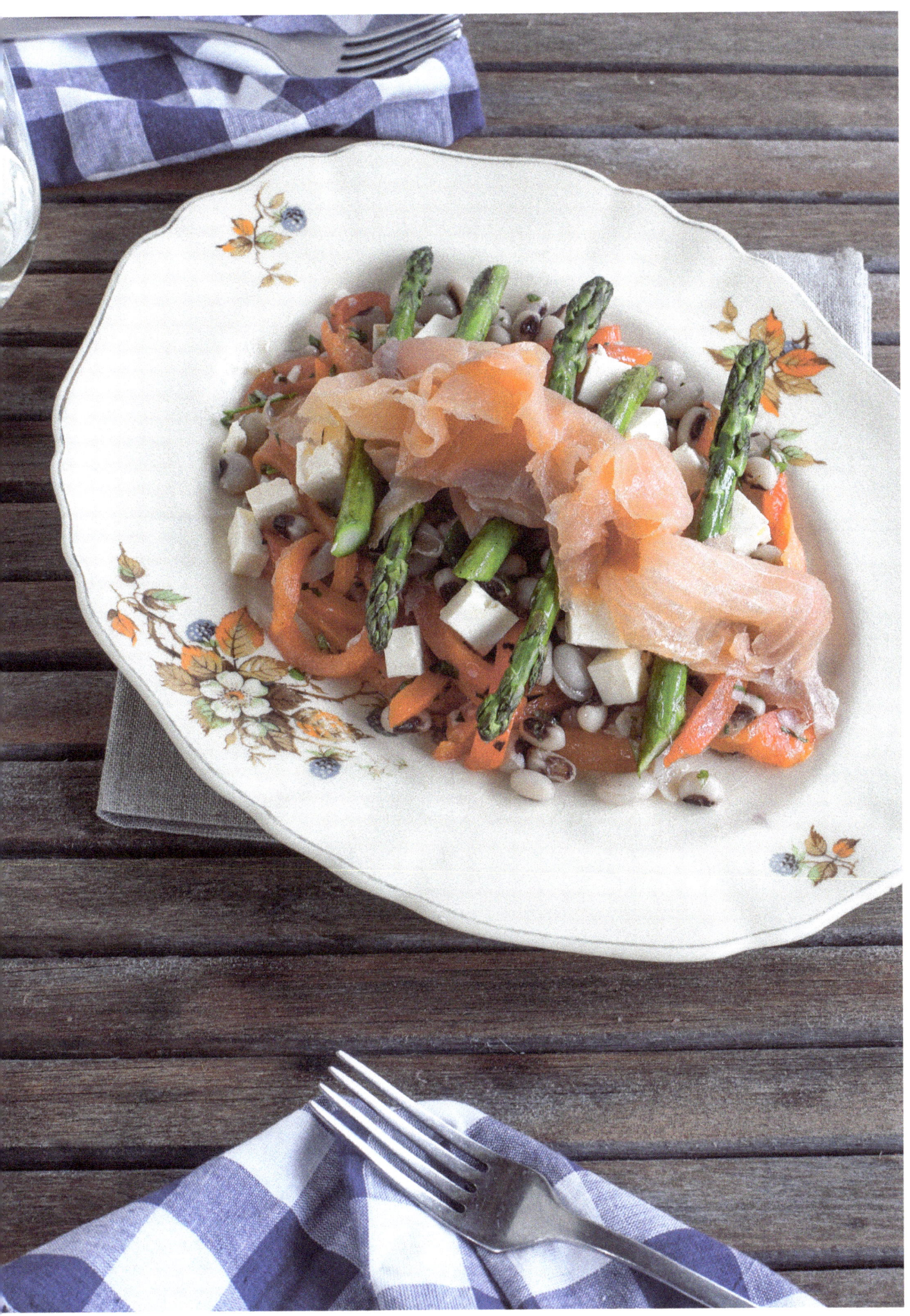

Family Salmon Casserole

SERVES 4-6

This recipe is a family favourite at my house. It is simple, super tasty, and can be made in advance. You can substitute tuna for the salmon and it is easily made from pantry staples.

CASSEROLE

25 grams butter

1 onion

2 cloves garlic

3 carrots

100 grams flour

500ml milk

1 teaspoon thyme

1 tablespoon tarragon

1 tablespoon parsley

100 grams cheddar cheese

1 cup peas (fresh, frozen or tinned)

1 cup corn (fresh, frozen or tinned)

400 grams salmon (tinned, smoked or fresh)

2 cups cooked pasta
(see page 30 to make your own)

CRUMB TOPPING

50 grams parmesan cheese

4 slices bread

1 tablespoon butter

1 teaspoon ground fennel

salt and pepper

Pre-heat the oven to 180°C.

To make the casserole, melt the butter in a heavy-based frying pan over medium heat. Finely dice the onion, crush the garlic, add to the pan and sauté.

Peel and finely dice the carrots, add to the pan and continue to sauté for 2 minutes. Add the flour and cook for a further 2 minutes, stirring well to cook the flour.

Slowly add the milk whilst continuing to stir. Bring the mixture to the boil, reduce heat to a simmer, and stir until the sauce has thickened. This will take 5 to 10 minutes.

Finely chop the thyme, tarragon and parsley, grate the cheese and add to the sauce along with the peas, corn salmon and cooked pasta. Add the remaining ingredients and stir to combine. Tip into a large casserole dish.

Use a food processor to make the crumb topping. Roughly chop the bread and parmesan cheese and process to a fine crumb. Add the butter, fennel, salt and pepper to taste, and process to combine. Spread evenly on top of the casserole.

Bake for 20 minutes, or until the crumb topping is golden brown.

Serve with a crisp green salad.

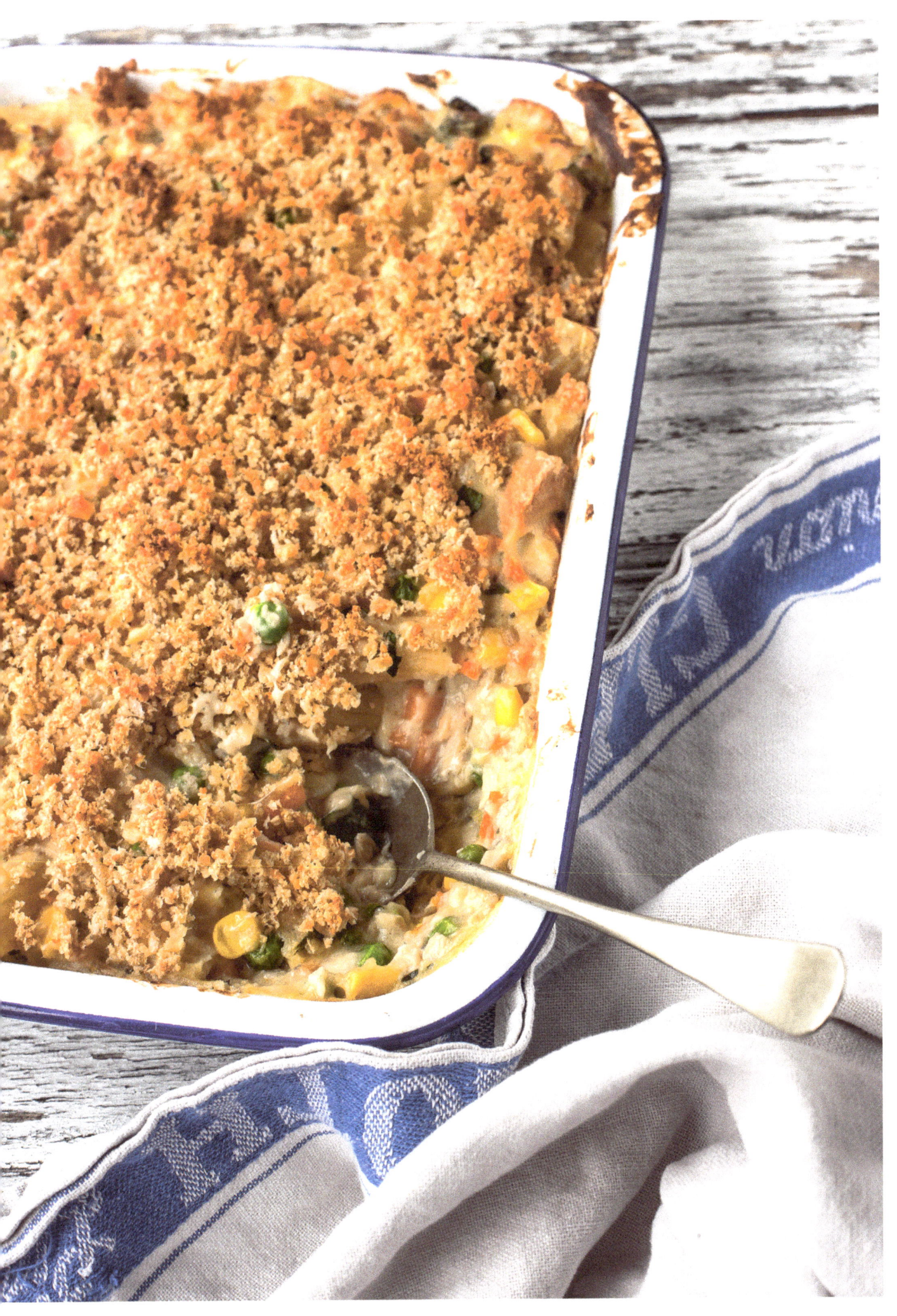

Caper Tart with Smoked Salmon and Red Onion Jam

SERVES 6

This tart tastes fabulous with its rich, homemade shortcrust pastry but to save time you can substitute 4 frozen sheets of shortcrust pastry instead. These tarts are delicious served hot or cold.

8 slices smoked salmon

PASTRY TART BASE

2 cups flour

¼ teaspoon salt

125 grams butter

1 egg

1 tablespoon water

TART FILLING

100 grams Gruyere cheese

1 teaspoon garlic

1 teaspoon tarragon

1 tablespoon capers

1 tablespoon chopped onion

5 eggs

1 cup cream

RED ONION JAM

1 teaspoon extra virgin olive oil

4 Spanish onions

¼ cup brown sugar

¼ cup caster sugar

¼ cup red wine vinegar

Use a food processor to make the pastry. Put flour and salt in the processor, add the cubed butter and blend until the mixture forms fine crumbs. With the motor running, add the egg then slowly add enough cold water to bring the dough together. Roll out the pastry to approximately 4 mm thick and line 6 small tart tins. Place the tins in the refrigerator to rest for at least ½ hour.

To make the tart filling, pre-heat the oven to 175°C. Grate the Gruyere cheese, crush the garlic, chop the tarragon and capers, dice the onion and mix well with the eggs and cream. Pour the filling into the tart cases and bake for 25 minutes or until cooked and golden brown

To make the red onion jam, heat the extra virgin olive oil in a heavy-based saucepan over medium heat, slice the onions, add to the pan and sweat for a few minutes, or until cooked. Add the sugars and vinegar and simmer for ½ hour. Set aside to cool.

Serve the tarts warm, hot or cold topped with smoked salmon and a generous dollop of the onion jam.

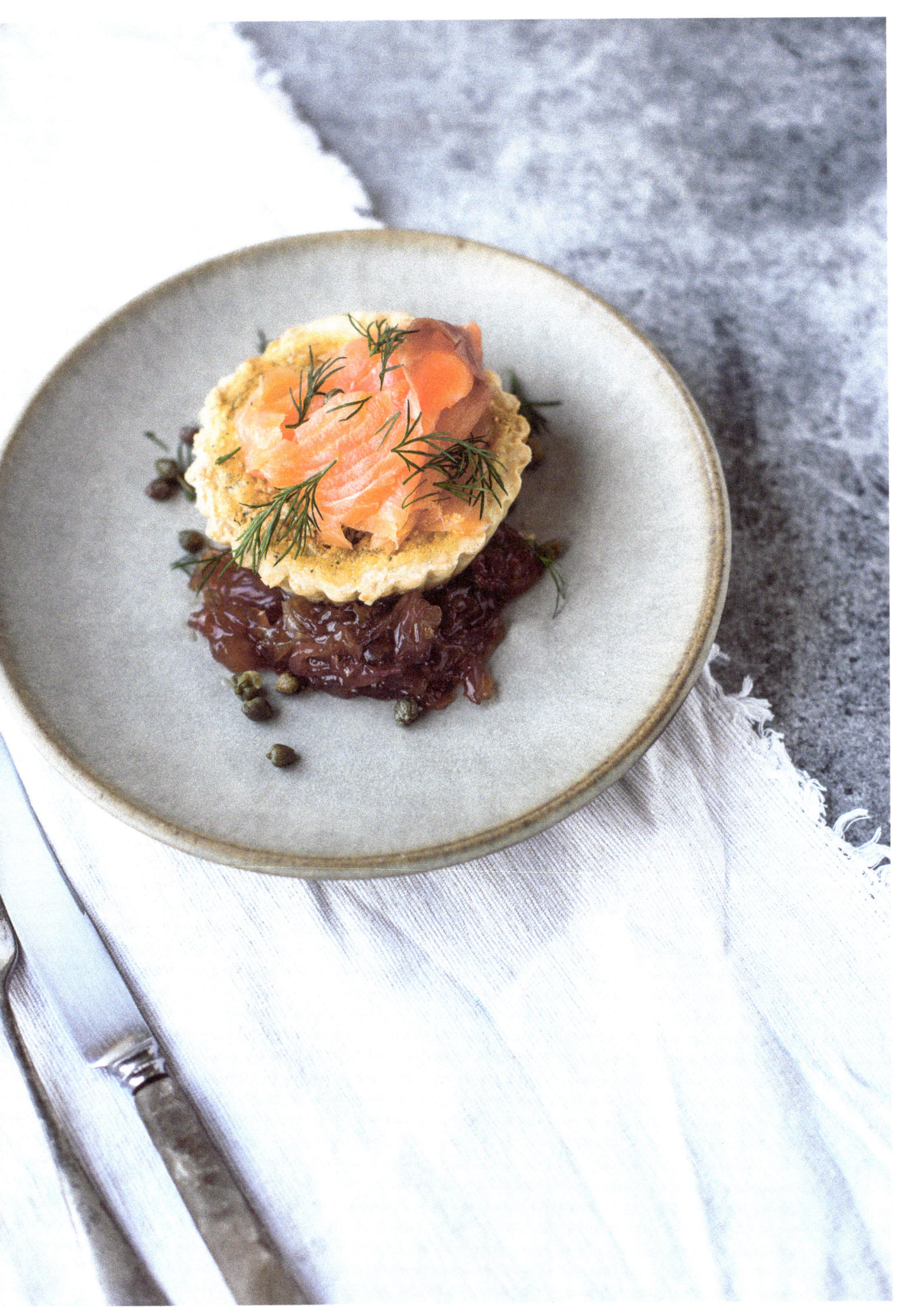

Salmon Rashers with French Toast and Maple Syrup

SERVES 4 FOR BREAKFAST

Salmon rashers are strips of salmon that have been smoked and sliced ready to grill, and are a great alternative to bacon.

2 eggs

½ cup milk

salt and pepper

extra virgin olive oil spray

400 grams (or 8) salmon rashers

4 thick slices bread

1 tablespoon butter

4 tablespoons maple syrup

Pre-heat the flat grill plate of the barbeque, or a frying pan on the stove top, over a low heat.

Whisk the eggs and milk together in a bowl, and season with a little salt and pepper.

Spray the barbeque with extra virgin olive oil spray and place the salmon rashers on the hottest part of the grill plate. Cook for a few minutes on each side, or until crisp.

Dip a slice of bread into the egg mixture, letting the bread soak up the mix for a few seconds on each side.

Cut the butter into four equal pieces. Place a lump of butter on the barbeque (in a cooler spot) and put the bread on top. Repeat with the other slices.

Cook the bread for two minutes on each side or until golden brown.

Serve the French toast with salmon rashers and a drizzle of maple syrup.

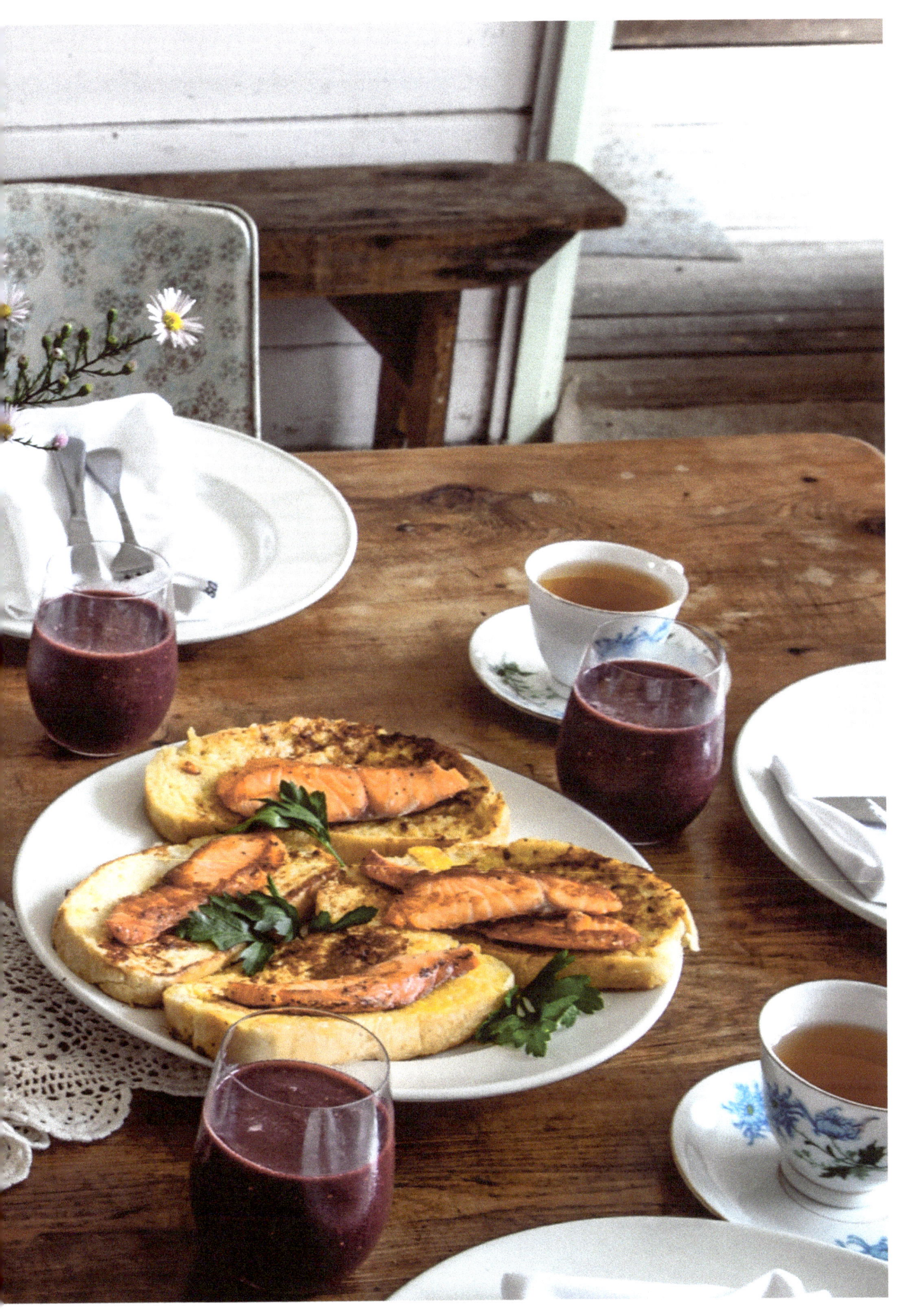

Dill and Feta Omelette

SERVES 4

1 clove garlic

2 tablespoons fresh dill

100 grams feta cheese

8 eggs

100 grams cream

salt and pepper

20 grams butter

200 grams smoked salmon

Crush the garlic, finely chop the dill and crumble the feta cheese. Whisk together the eggs and cream in a large bowl, add the garlic, dill and feta, and whisk to combine. Season with salt and pepper.

Melt the butter in a large frying pan over medium heat, pour in the egg mixture and cook for 10 minutes or until the omelette is set.

Serve hot, warm or cold topped with the smoked salmon and dill.

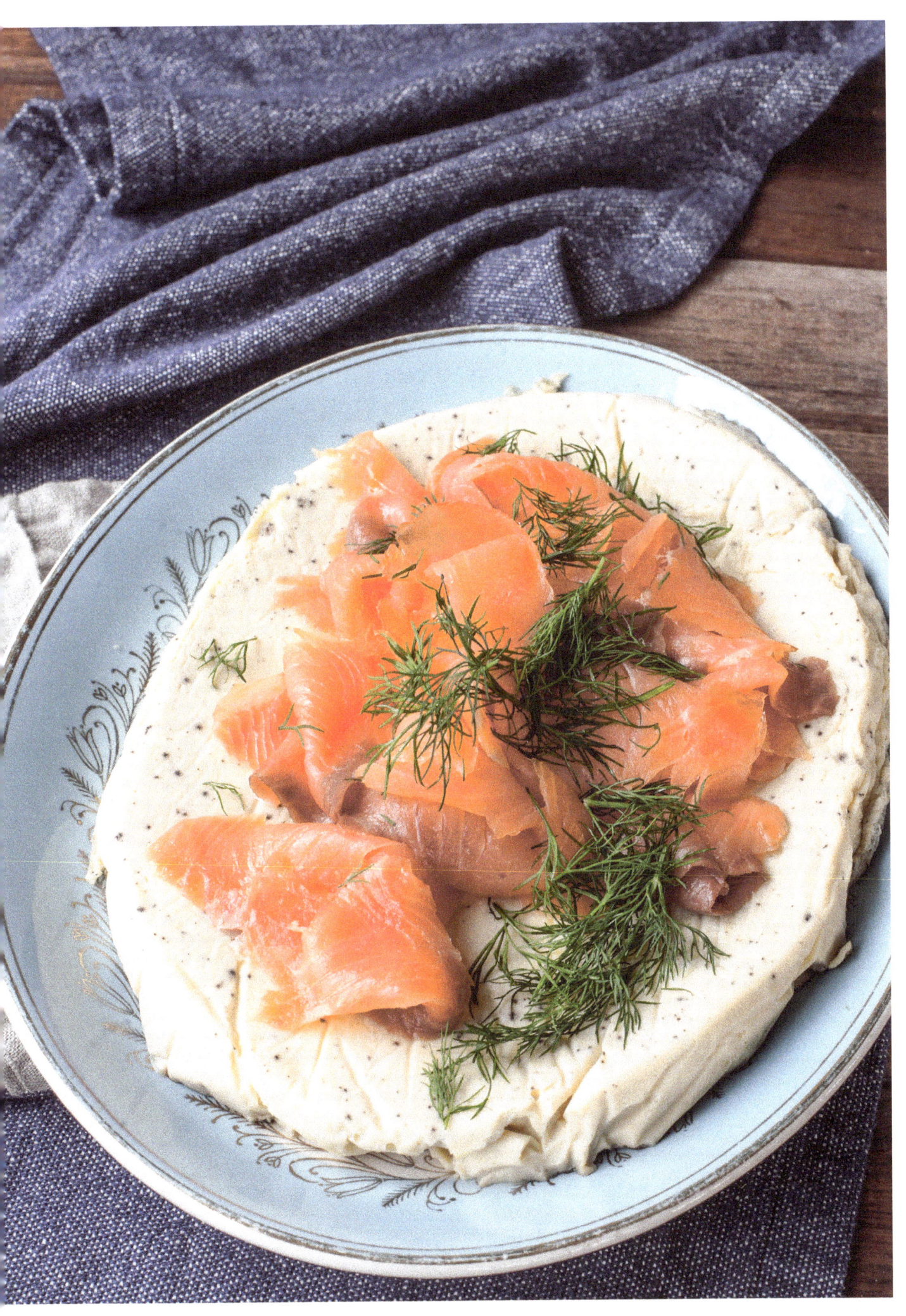

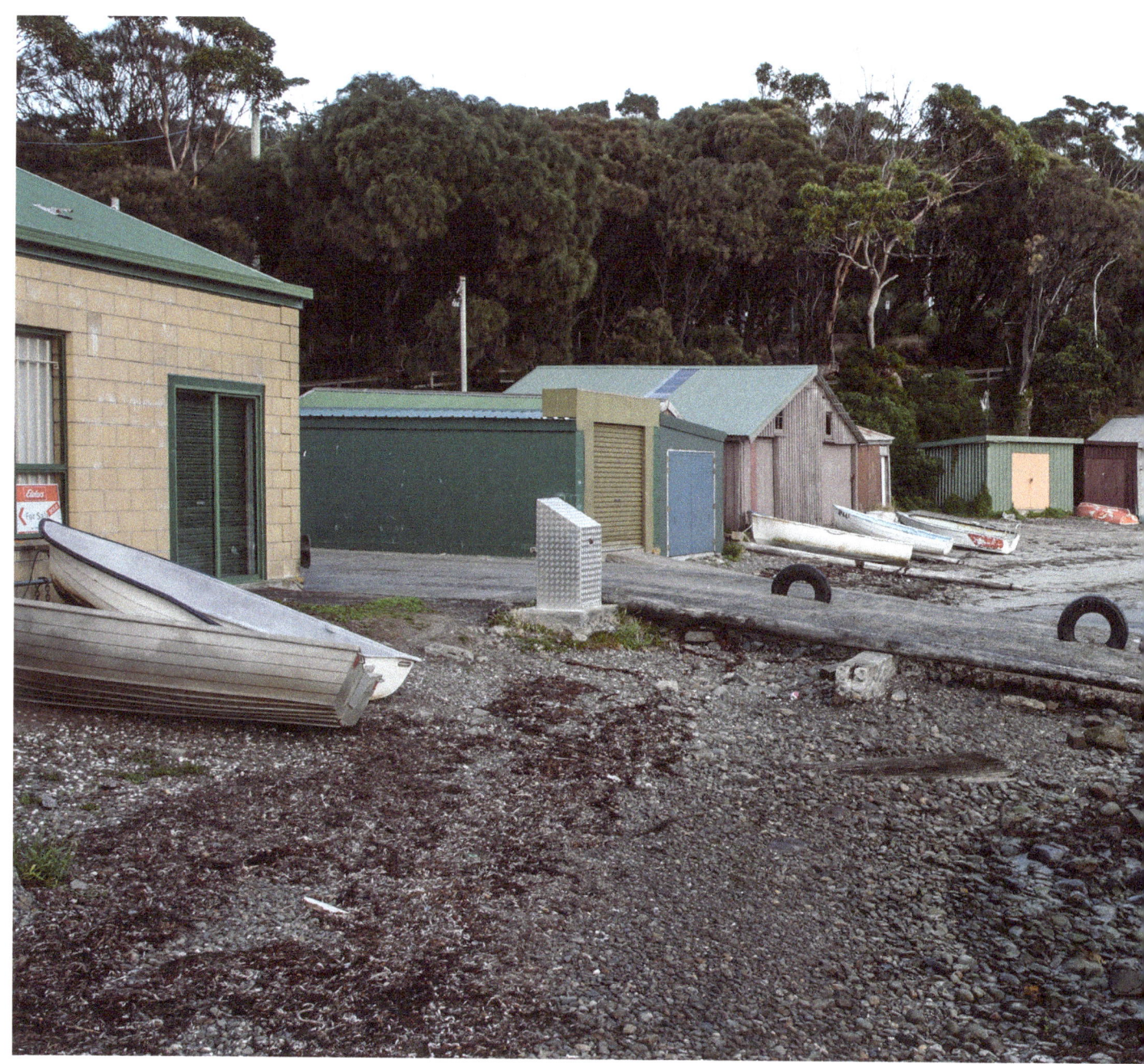

Economical Fish Meals

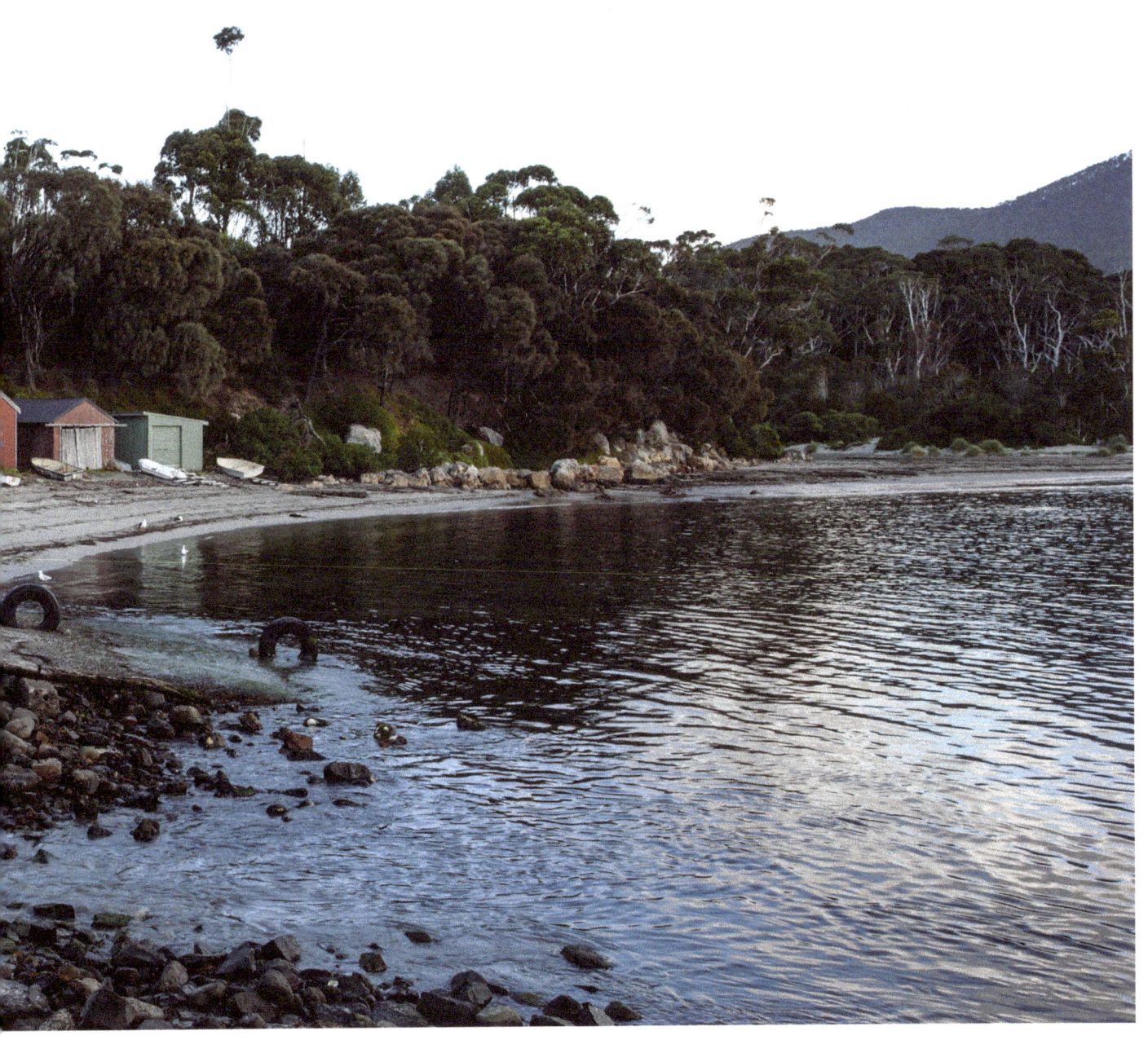

Laksa

SERVES 4-6

The bold, punchy flavours of freshly made laksa paste make this a stand out dish, and the quantity given here makes more paste than you will need for one recipe. To store the remaining paste, pour into a jar and top with a little extra virgin olive oil. Alternatively, freeze tablespoons in ice-cube trays and store the frozen cubes in a zip-lock bag for months. You can also use a jar of ready-made laksa paste. Although I have used seafood here you could substitute chicken or mixed veggies for a vegetarian option. If some of the mussels don't open during the cooking time, don't throw them out, they are still good to eat. Simply open them with the tip of a knife.

PASTE

1 small red onion

½ knob ginger

1 stalk lemongrass

½ tablespoon shrimp paste

1 lime

4 dried birds-eye chillies

1 teaspoon coriander seed

1 teaspoon turmeric

6 cloves garlic

1 teaspoon ginger

½ bunch coriander

1 tablespoon basil

5 kaffir lime leaves

50ml extra virgin olive oil

LAKSA

50ml extra virgin olive oil

800 grams mussels

300 grams white fish

1 squid tube and legs

2 cups fresh greens, such as bok choy or spinach

2 cups rice noodles

1 onion

500ml fish stock

500ml coconut cream

red chilli to garnish

coriander to garnish

To make the laksa paste, roughly chop the onion, ginger and white part of the lemongrass, zest and juice the lime, and place into a food processor, along with all remaining paste ingredients. Blend well, until a smooth paste has formed.

Cook the noodles following the directions on the packet, and set aside until needed.

De-beard and clean mussels if necessary. Cut the fish into 2cm pieces. Clean the squid by removing the skin and cartilage, cut the tube through one side to lay it down flat on a chopping board. Using a sharp knife, cut the flesh lightly halfway through in a criss-cross pattern with scores on an angle about 5 mm apart. Roughly chop the greens and set aside.

Heat a wok over high heat, add the squid and sear for about 1 minute, remove and set aside. Reheat the wok to a high heat and add the extra virgin olive oil and sauté the sliced onions for a few minutes or until softened. Add the mussels, fish and 2 tablespoons of laksa paste, and cook stirring, for one minute.

Add the stock and coconut cream, bring to a simmer and cook until the mussels start to open.

Toss through the noodles, squid and greens and serve immediately topped with freshly sliced chilli and coriander leaves.

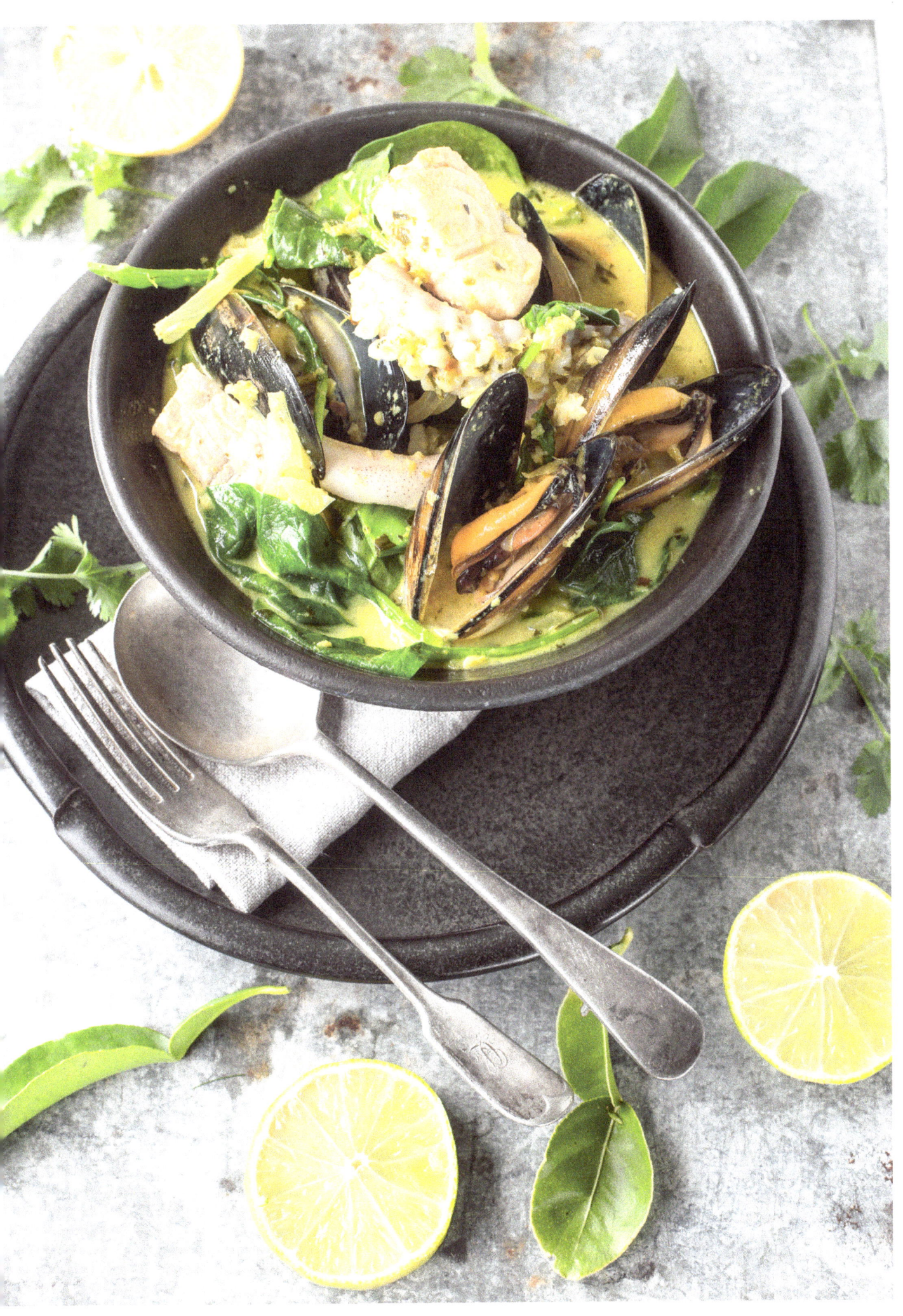

Spicy Fish Tortillas

SERVES 4-6

Making tortilla dough is easy and satisfying, and homemade tortillas taste wonderful. If you are pressed for time however, shop-bought tortillas are a good alternative. Kids love to create and wrap their own tortillas and you can reduce or remove the cayenne and chilli from the recipe if you want a milder flavour. You can make the tortilla dough a few hours in advance, but be sure to wrap it very well in plastic wrap to avoid it drying out and store in the refrigerator.

TORTILLAS

¾ cup milk

2 cups self raising flour

1 ½ teaspoon baking powder

1 teaspoon salt

2 teaspoons extra virgin olive oil

extra virgin olive oil spray

SLAW

⅛ green cabbage

3 big spring onions

1 bunch coriander

2 limes

1 lemon

SPICY FISH

5 tablespoons flour

½ teaspoon salt

½ teaspoon cayenne pepper

¼ teaspoon chilli

¼ teaspoon tumeric

¼ teaspoon cumin

¼ teaspoon coriander

600 grams boneless skinless fish fillets

2 tablespoons extra virgin olive oil

200ml sour cream to serve

To make the tortillas, warm the milk slightly and mix in a bowl with the flour, baking powder, salt and extra virgin olive oil until well combined.

Knead the dough on a floured board for a few minutes or until smooth. Cover the dough with plastic wrap and rest for 20 minutes.

Divide the dough into 8 equal portions and rest for a further 10 minutes. Roll each portion into a round about 1.5mm in thickness.

Heat a frying pan over low heat and brush lightly with extra virgin olive oil (or use oil spray), place a tortilla into the pan and cook for one minute on each side. Repeat for remaining tortillas. Keep tortillas warm until required by wrapping in foil and placing in a low oven.

To make the slaw, finely slice the cabbage, spring onions and coriander and combine in a large bowl. Juice the lemon and limes, and pour juice over the slaw.

To cook the fish, place the flour, salt and all the spices into a freezer bag and shake well to combine. Cut the fish into 1cm wide strips, add to the bag and shake well to coat. Heat the extra virgin olive oil in a heavy based frying pan over medium heat and cook the fish strips for 2 minutes on each side or until golden brown and cooked through.

To serve, top each tortilla with slaw, fish and sour cream and wrap firmly.

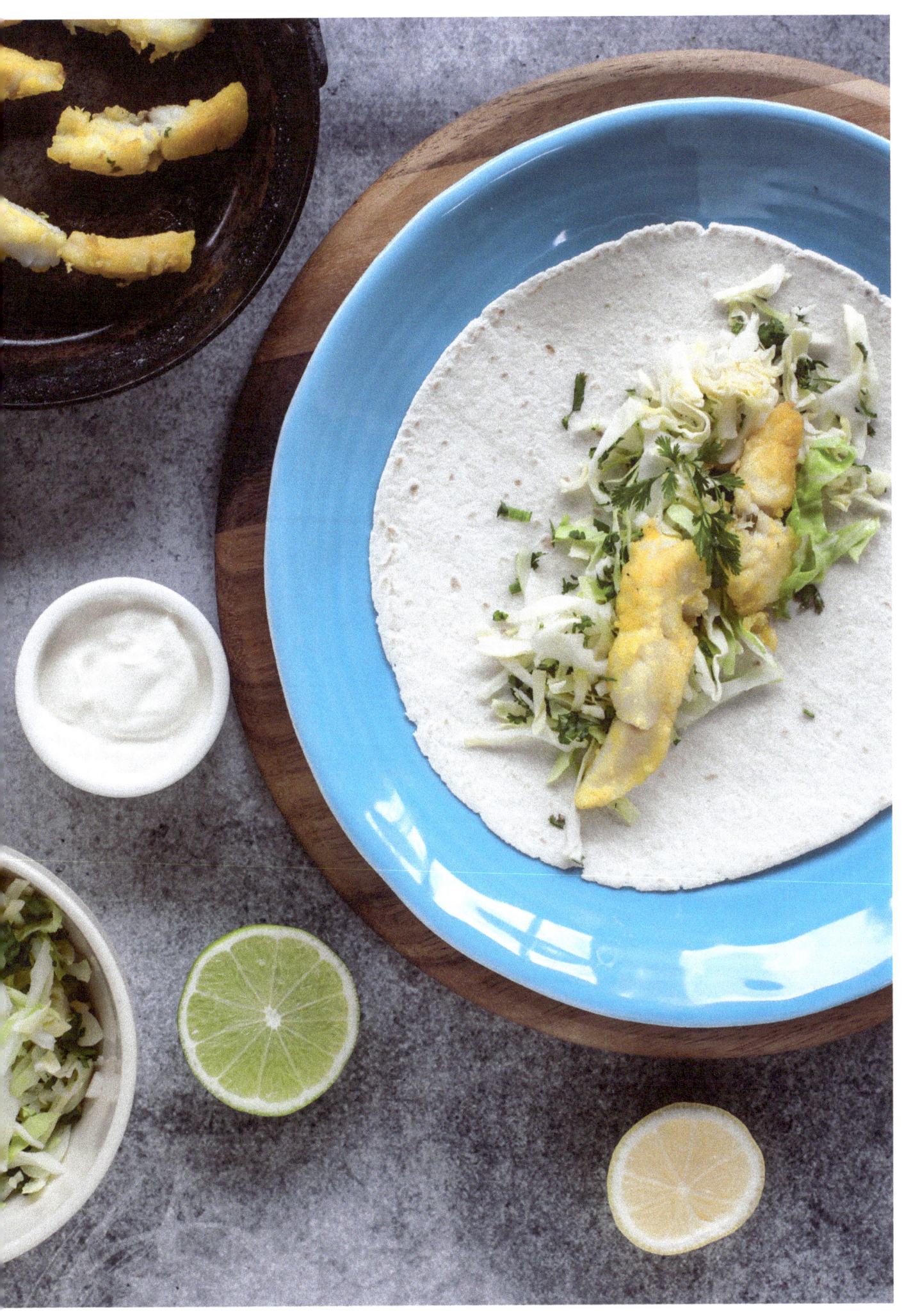

Fish Chowder

SERVES 4

I like to use Bay Trumpeter in this recipe, but you could use any fish you like in this creamy and filling soup. It is delicious served with crusty bread and butter, or warm bread rolls.

1 onion

1 carrot

5 cloves garlic

1 tablespoon tarragon

2 tablespoons dill

40 grams butter

salt and pepper

¾ cups plain flour

750ml fish stock

100ml white wine

500ml milk

250ml cream

500 grams white-fleshed fish

80 grams parmesan cheese

Peel and dice the onion and carrot, crush the garlic and finely chop the tarragon and dill. Using a heavy-based saucepan, melt the butter over low heat and sauté the onion, carrot, garlic, tarragon and add salt and pepper to taste.

Add flour and cook, stirring, for 2 minutes. Add the stock and wine, and continue to cook over a low heat until the carrot is tender. Add the milk and cream and gently return to the boil, taking care not to overheat, as this will scald the milk.

Dice the fish into 2cm cubes. Once at a gentle boil, add the diced fish and simmer for a few minutes or until the fish is cooked through. Add the grated parmesan cheese and serve.

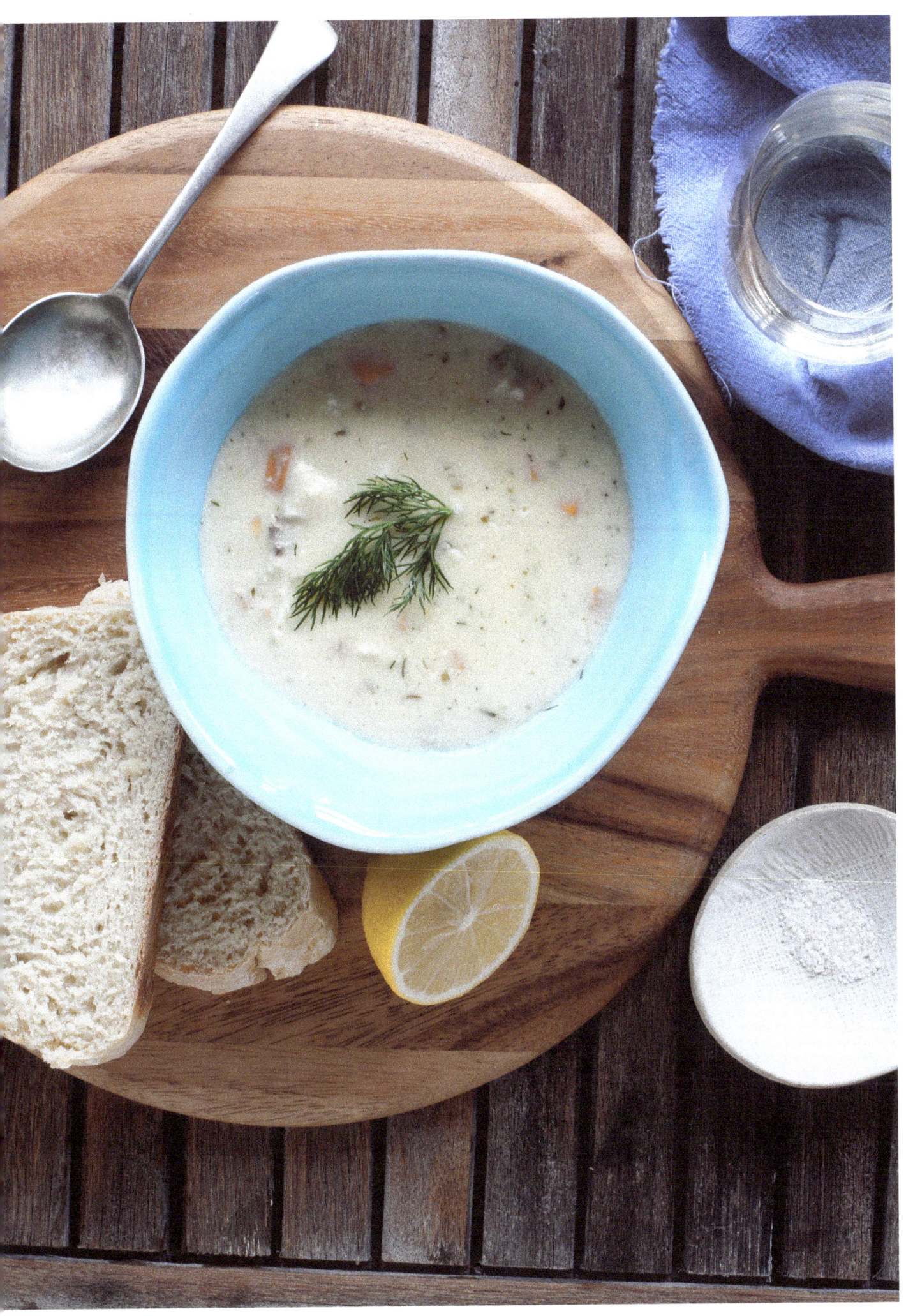

Fish Lasagna with Fennel and Tarragon

SERVES 6

It is best to use a flaky, white-fleshed fish for this lasagna, such as Bay Trumpeter or Australian Salmon. The fresh pasta has a luxurious, tender texture and makes this a special dish, however ready-made lasagna sheets may be substituted for the fresh pasta. Serve the lasagna with a crisp green salad in summer, or some sautéed green beans and spinach when the weather gets cooler.

FRESH PASTA

200 grams flour

2 eggs

FISH SAUCE

2 onions

4 cloves garlic

1 tablespoon extra virgin olive oil

800 grams tomatoes

½ teaspoon ground fennel

1 tablespoon basil

1 tablespoon tarragon

1 tablespoon oregano

600 grams fresh fish

CHEESE SAUCE

2 tablespoons butter

2 tablespoons plain flour

500ml milk

100 grams cheddar cheese

50 grams parmesan cheese

salt and pepper

Preheat the oven to 180°C.

To make the pasta, put the flour into a large bowl and make a well in the centre. Add the eggs to the flour and combine until a smooth dough is formed. Turn out onto a clean surface or board and knead well for at least 5 minutes, or until the pasta is smooth. Divide the dough into 4 smaller portions. Using a pasta machine set at number 1 (or at the widest setting) feed the dough through the pasta machine in small batches. Repeat this process 3-4 more times, increasing the setting each time until the pasta is approximately 2mm thick and silky smooth. Dust the bench with flour and carefully lay dough aside until needed.

To make the fish sauce, dice the onions and crush the garlic. Using a heavy based pan, heat the extra virgin olive oil over moderate heat and sauté the onion and garlic until soft. Roughly chop the tomatoes, finely chop the herbs and add to the sauce along with the fennel. Simmer for 20 minutes, stirring occasionally. Dice fish into 2 cm pieces, add to the tomato sauce and simmer for a few minutes until the fish is just cooked and can be easily flaked apart.

To make the cheese sauce, melt the butter in a heavy based saucepan, add the flour and stir until combined. Gradually add the milk and bring to a simmer, stirring continuously, until the sauce is thick and smooth. Grate the cheeses, stir through the sauce and season to taste with salt and pepper.

To form the lasagna, lightly grease a baking dish or tray. Spoon a layer of fish mixture into the tray to create an even layer, top with the pasta sheets and continue until all of the mixture is used. Finish with a layer of pasta and top with the cheese sauce.

Bake for 30 minutes or until the top is golden brown and the pasta sheets are cooked through.

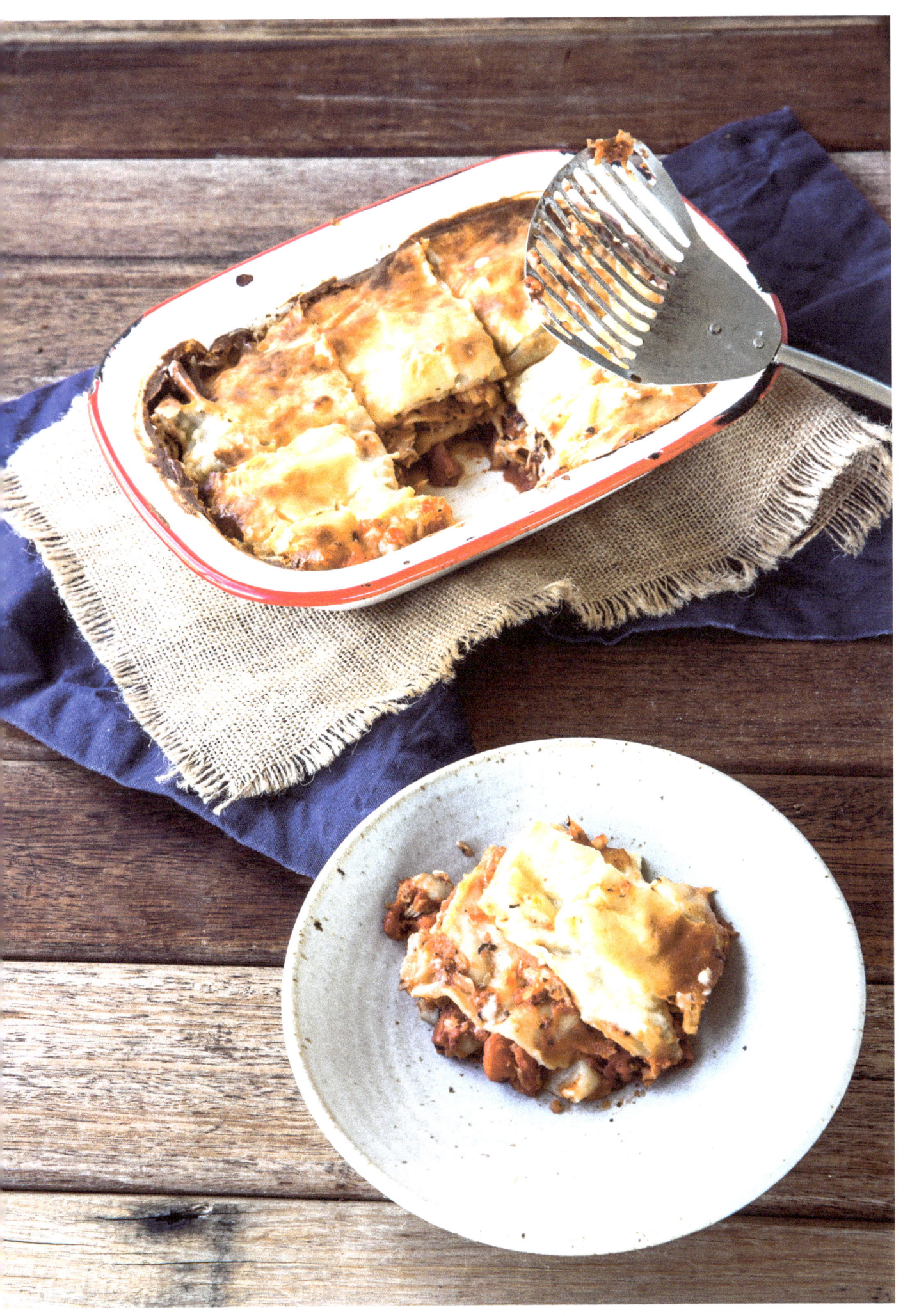

Fish Pie

SERVES 4

This is a delicious, warming winter dish. You can use any white-fleshed fish in the filling, or frozen fish would also be a good alternative. If you want to add few veggies, simply include peas, beans or spinach to the fish mixture. Serve the pie with garden salad and chutney, and add some crusty bread for hungry family and friends.

PASTRY

200 grams plain flour

salt

100 grams butter

50ml water

PIE FILLING

1 brown onion

1 leek, white part only

2 cloves garlic

1 tablespoon butter

60 grams flour

300ml milk

100ml cream

500 grams white-fleshed fish (skin and bones removed)

1 tablespoon tarragon

60 grams parmesan cheese

1 teaspoon ground fennel seed

sea salt and cracked black pepper

TOPPING

2 cups mashed potato, cooled (recipe page 110)

60 grams cheddar cheese

To make the pastry, place the flour and salt into a bowl, chop the cold butter into pieces and rub the butter into the flour with your fingers, until the mixture resembles fine crumbs. Mix the water into the crumb mixture until the dough has come together, and then knead on a floured bench until the pastry feels smooth.

Alternatively, make the pastry in the food processor. Place flour and diced cold butter into the processor, pulse until the mixture resembles fine crumbs, and slowly add the water with the motor running, until the dough comes together. Wrap the dough in plastic wrap and set aside to rest for at least half an hour. The dough can be rested on the bench if you are planning on rolling it out straight away, otherwise rest it in the fridge and bring back to room temperature before rolling.

Pre-heat the oven to 180°C. Roll the pastry out to a thickness of 5mm and line the base and sides of a 20cm pie dish, or 4 individual pie dishes. To blind bake the pastry, bake the pastry-lined tins for 20 minutes or until golden and cooked through.

To make the pie filling, finely dice the onion and leek, and crush the garlic. Melt the butter in a heavy-based saucepan over medium heat and sauté the onion, leek and garlic for 3 minutes or until soft. Add the flour and cook for 2 minutes. Add the milk and cream whilst stirring and bring to a simmer. Continue to simmer until the sauce has started to thicken. Chop the fish and tarragon, grate the cheese and add to the sauce along with the ground fennel and season with salt and pepper. Reduce the heat to low and simmer for a few minutes or until the fish is just cooked (or slightly undercooked – the fish will finish cooking when reheated).

Pour the filling into the pastry case. Spread the mashed potato over the top of the fish mixture, grate the cheese and sprinkle it over the potato topping. The pie can now be refrigerated until you are ready to cook and serve.

When you are ready to cook the pie, preheat the oven to 180°C and cook for about 20 minutes to heat through the pie and brown the potato topping.

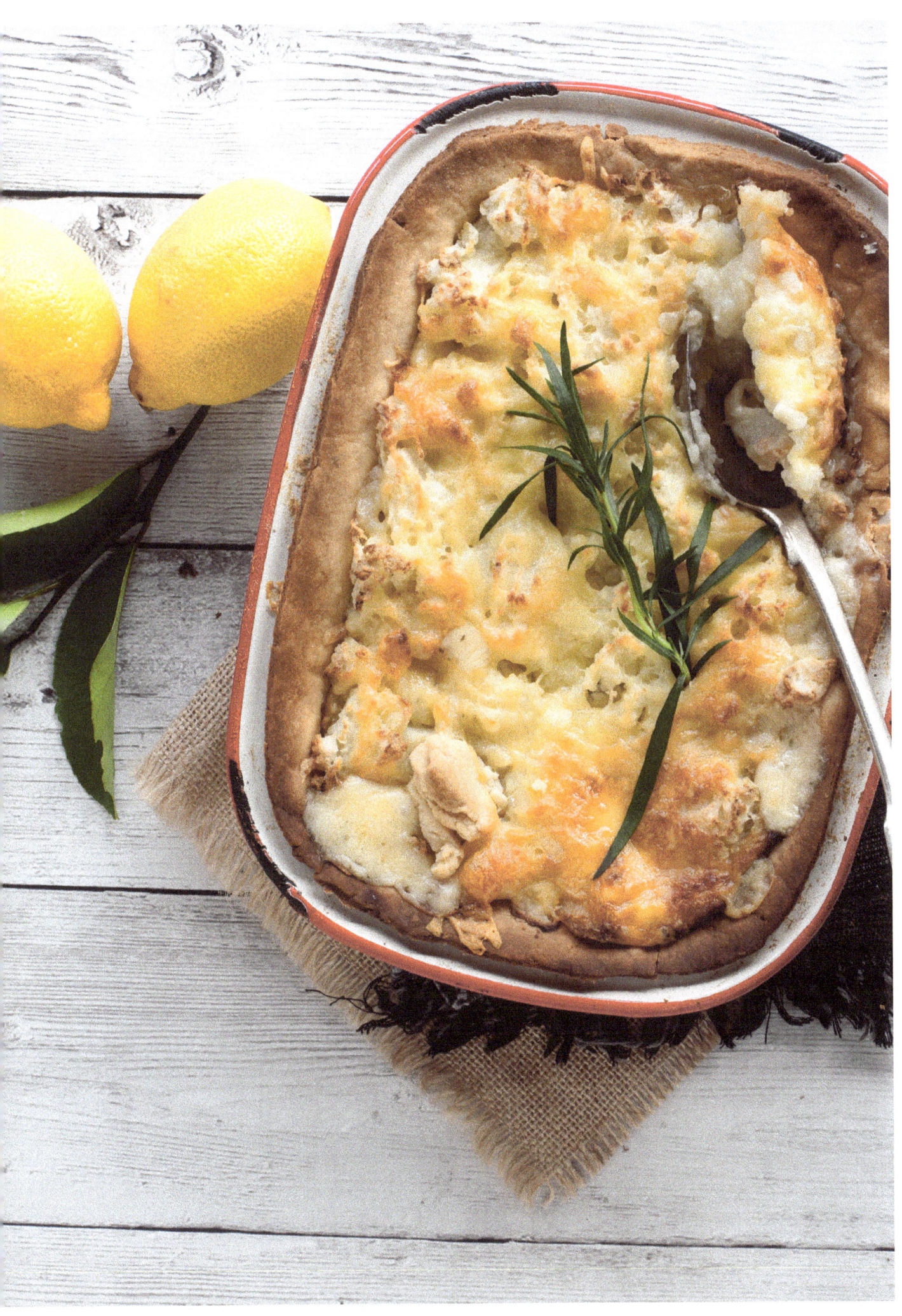

Moroccan Seafood Stew

SERVES 4

The sauce for this scrumptious fish stew can be easily made in advance and is even better when pre-prepared, as it allows the flavours plenty of time to develop. Once the sauce is made, this is a simple and delicious meal to whip up on a busy weeknight. Use any seafood you like for this stew. Preserved lemon is a wonderful ingredient that adds a complex flavor to dishes. A jar of preserved lemon will last for ages and is an extremely versatile ingredient to have on hand. To make your own preserved lemon visit www.eloiseemmett.com.

FISH STEW

1 medium onion

2 cloves garlic

1 teaspoon extra virgin olive oil

¼ teaspoon chilli flakes

1 teaspoon crushed fennel seed

½ teaspoon crushed coriander seed

½ teaspoon ground ginger

1 teaspoon ground cumin

½ teaspoon sweet paprika

⅛ of a preserved lemon (or 1 teaspoon, chopped)

300ml vegetable or fish stock

400 grams crushed tomatoes

600 grams white-fleshed fish

300 grams mussels

COUSCOUS

1 ½ cups vegetable stock

1 ½ cups couscous

1 tablespoon butter

½ a medium bunch coriander

To make the sauce for the stew, slice the onion and crush the garlic. Using a large frying pan, heat the extra virgin olive oil over medium heat and sauté the onion and garlic for a few minutes, or until the onion has softened. Add the chilli flakes, fennel and coriander seed, ginger, cumin and paprika and cook, stirring, for 2 minutes. Finely chop the preserved lemon and add to the pan, along with the stock and tomatoes, and cook for 10 minutes, stirring occasionally. Set the sauce aside for at least half an hour for the flavours to infuse.

When you are ready to serve, dice the fish into 2cm cubes and clean or prepare the mussels if necessary. Bring the sauce back to a gentle simmer, add the diced fish and mussels, and continue to simmer for a further 5 minutes or until the seafood is cooked to your liking.

To prepare the couscous, bring the stock to the boil in a saucepan, sprinkle in the couscous, stir well and cover with a lid for 4 minutes. Remove the lid, add the butter and fluff the couscous with a fork.

Serve the fish stew with the couscous and sprinkle with fresh coriander.

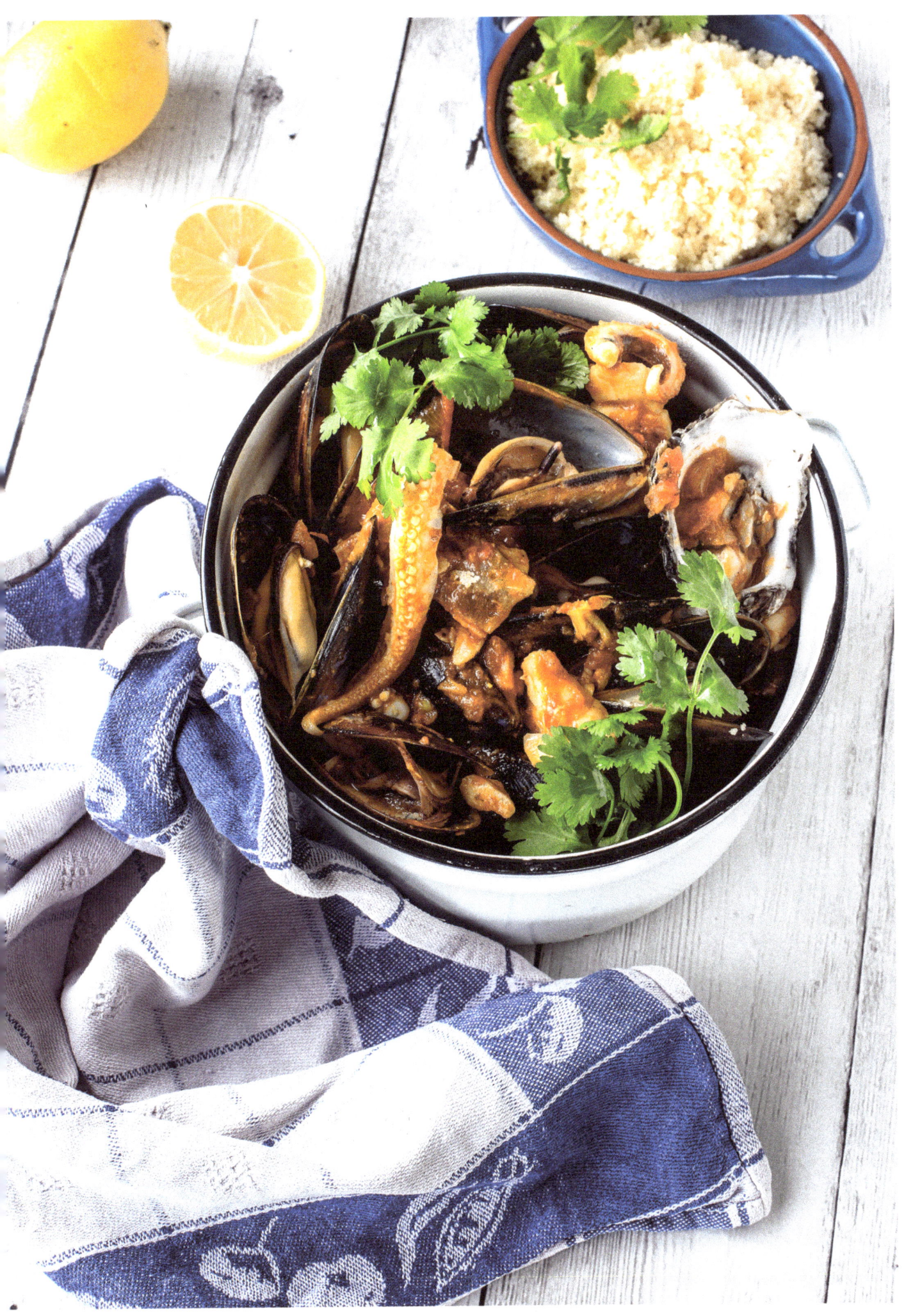

Fish Burgers

SERVES 4

Serve these burgers in a crusty bun with salad and tartare sauce for a tasty and healthy family meal. Use an economical, white-fleshed, flaky fish for these burgers, such as Bay Trumpeter.

2 large Kennebec potatoes

1 small sweet potato

400 grams fish

1 clove crushed garlic

2 wedges preserved lemon

2 tablespoons tarragon

1 tablespoon parsley

20 chives

1 egg

1 cup bread crumbs

TO SERVE

salad

tartare sauce

crusty bun

Peel and dice the Kennebec and sweet potatoes. Put potatoes into a large saucepan, cover with water, bring to the boil and cook for 15-20 minutes or until cooked through. Drain well, cool slightly and mash. Steam the fish by placing a bamboo steamer over boiling water and steaming for 2-3 minutes or until cooked.

Alternatively, the fish can be poached – fill a large saucepan with 5cm of water, bring to a simmer, add the fish and poach for 2-3 minutes or until cooked. Crush the garlic, finely dice the preserved lemon and herbs, and mix into the mashed potato. Stir in the egg and season with salt and pepper. Roll into eight balls, flatten into patties and roll in the breadcrumbs.

Heat the extra virgin olive oil in a large heavy-based pan over medium heat, or on the flat grill of the BBQ, and fry for about 4 minutes on each side until golden and crispy.

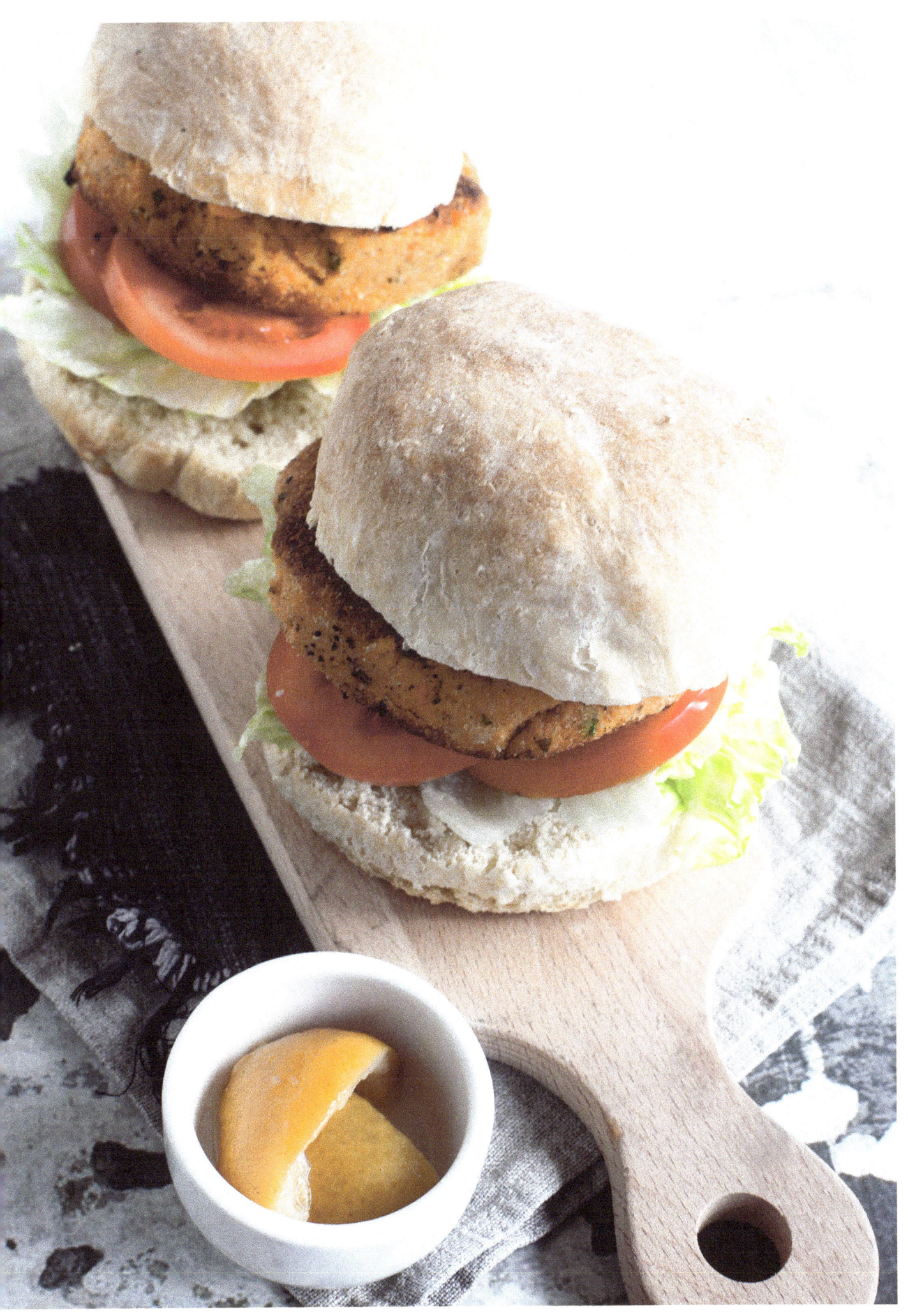

Tomato and Tarragon Seafood Broth

SERVES 4

This broth is very versatile. It can be used to flavour seafood risotto (see page 78) or may be served on its own as a soup. For a main meal, you can poach your preferred seafood in this broth and serve with crusty bread and saffron aioli. For the fish offcuts, any bones, skin, prawn or cray shells can be used.

1 medium onion

2 tomatoes (or 100 grams crushed tomatoes)

1 tablespoon extra virgin olive oil

1 teaspoon garlic

½ teaspoon fennel seed

1 tablespoon dried tarragon

250 grams fish offcuts

1 ½ tablespoons tomato paste

¼ cup plain flour

½ cup lemon juice

½ cup white wine

1 litre water

salt and pepper

SAFFRON AIOLI

1 egg

30ml white vinegar

½ teaspoon saffron threads

1 clove garlic

salt and pepper

200ml extra virgin olive oil

To make the stock, roughly chop the onion and dice the tomatoes. Heat the extra virgin olive oil in a large saucepan over medium heat, add the onion, garlic, fennel seed and dried tarragon and fry for a few minutes, or until the garlic and onion has softened.

Add the tomatoes, fish offcuts, tomato paste and plain flour and continue to cook stirring, for a few minutes. Add the lemon juice, wine and water, bring to the boil and simmer for 25 minutes. Season with salt and pepper and set aside to allow the flavours to infuse for a few hours, before straining through a sieve.

Use a food processor to make the aioli. Blend the egg, vinegar, saffron threads, garlic and a sprinkle of salt and pepper until well amalgamated. With the motor still running, pour the extra virgin olive oil into the processor in a slow drizzle until the aioli is thick and creamy.

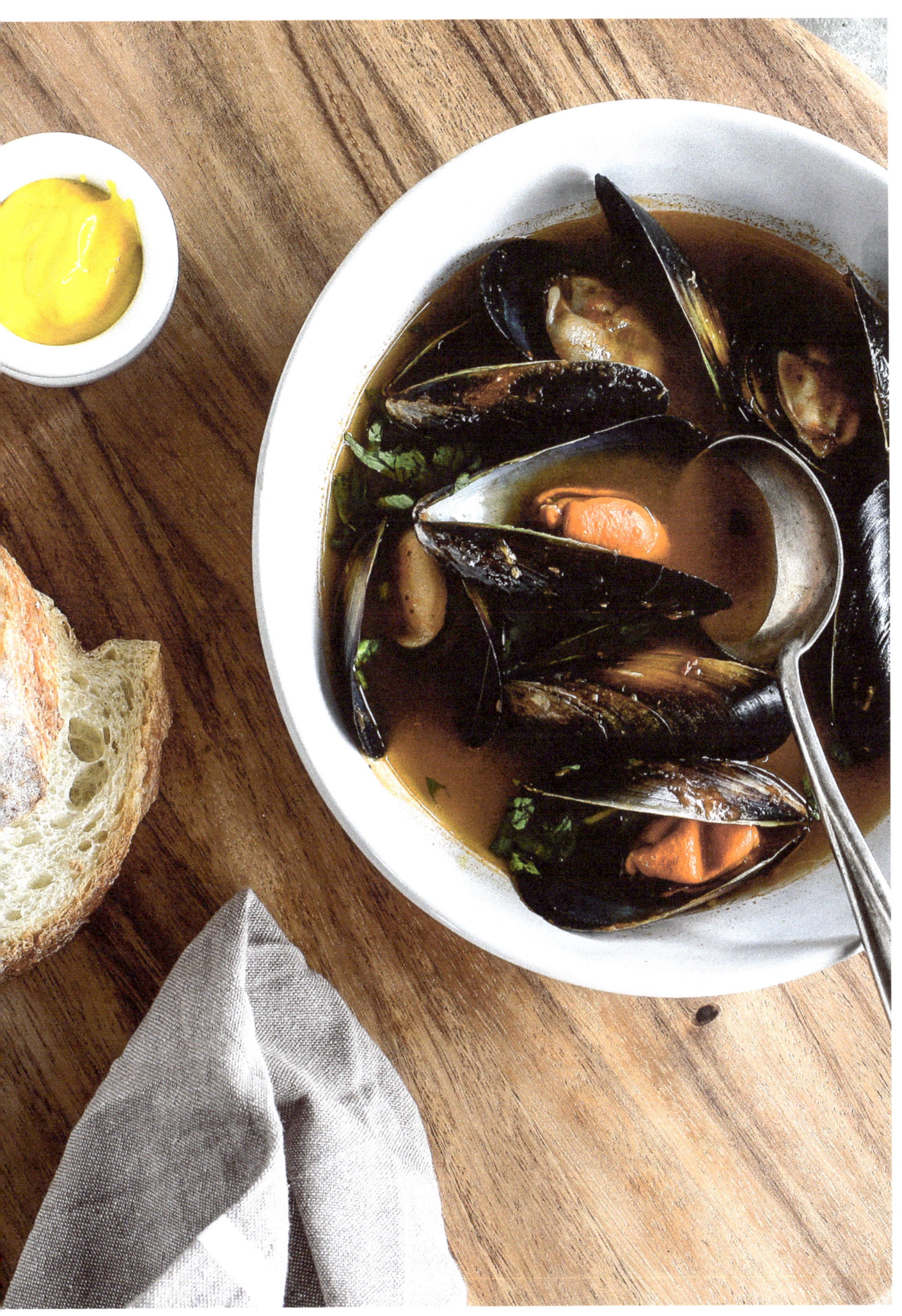

Seafood Risotto

SERVES 4

Timing is important in this dish. If you are using mussels, simply steam them in a separate pan in a little white wine and fold them through the cooked risotto before serving.

1 litre fish stock
(or use the broth recipe from page 76)

1 medium onion

2 cloves garlic

1 tablespoon butter

1 tablespoon extra virgin olive oil

300 grams Arborio rice

1 cup white wine

600 grams fish or seafood of your choice

50ml cream

1 cup spinach

½ cup parmesan

salt and pepper

To make the risotto, bring the stock to the boil in a saucepan, and then reduce the heat slightly to keep the stock at a slow boil.

Finely dice the onion and crush the garlic. In a large, heavy-based saucepan, melt the butter over medium heat, add the oil and sauté the onion and garlic for a few minutes, or until the onion is translucent.

Add the rice, reduce the heat to low and continue to sauté for 2 minutes. Increase to a medium heat, add the wine and one cup of hot stock, stirring continuously. When the liquid is almost absorbed, add another cup of the stock.

Continue to add the stock in this manner, until it is all used and the rice is very nearly cooked. This will take approximately 25 minutes.

Add the seafood and cream and continue stirring until the seafood and rice is cooked. Stir through the spinach and parmesan, season with salt and pepper and serve.

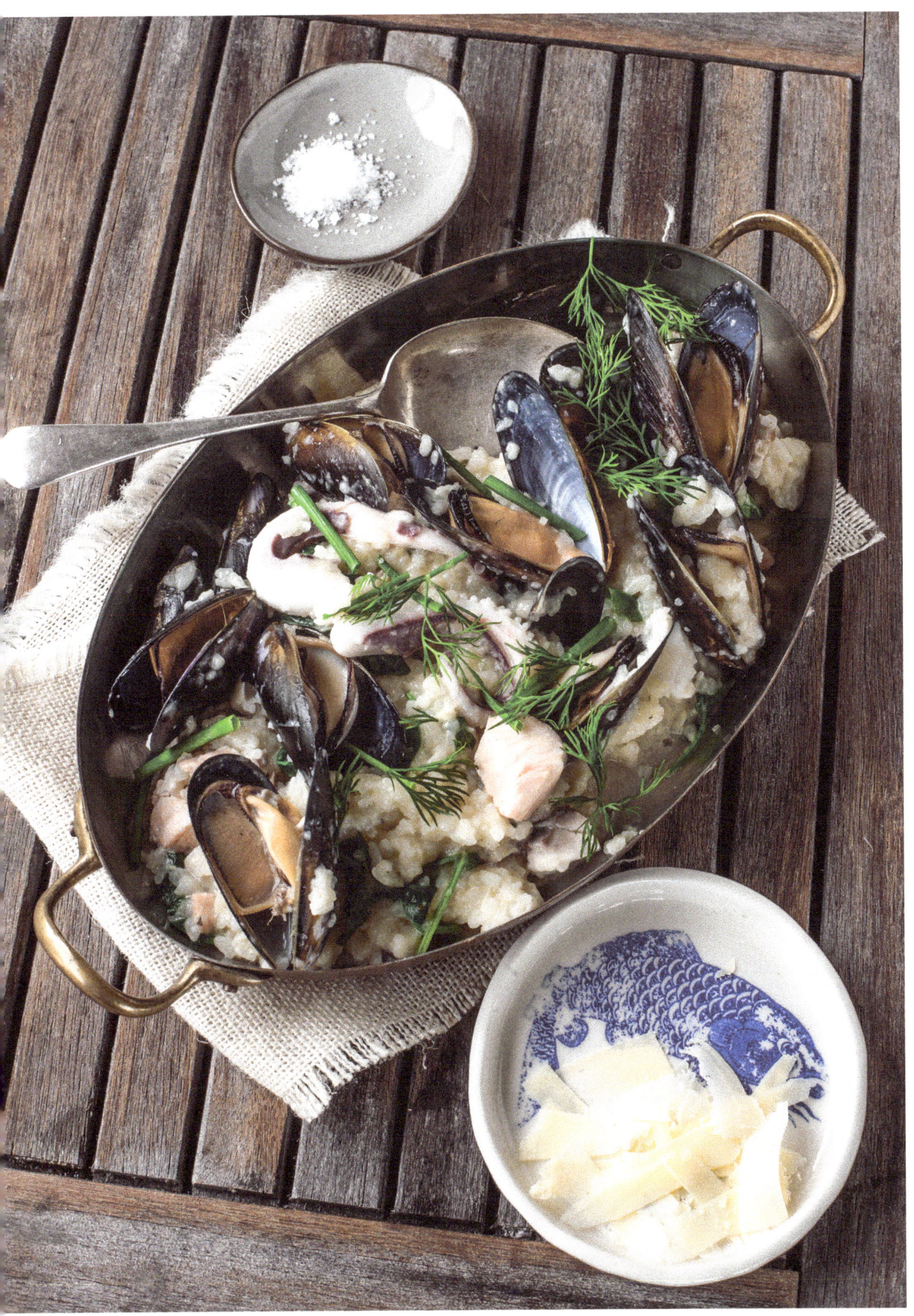

Honey Soy Marinated Fish and Asian Noodle Salad

SERVES 4

2 cloves garlic

2 tablespoons light soy sauce

1 tablespoon honey

1 tablespoon extra virgin olive oil

600 grams fish

3 tablespoons cornflour

2 tablespoons extra virgin olive oil

ASIAN SALAD DRESSING

1 tablespoon soy sauce

1 tablespoon white vinegar

1 teaspoon sugar

¼ cup extra virgin olive oil

1 tablespoon sesame oil

salt and pepper

ASIAN NOODLE SALAD

¼ cabbage

2 carrots

4 spring onions

1 cup noodles (cooked rice noodles, fried noodles or mixture of both)

To prepare the fish, crush the garlic and mix with the soy, honey and 1 tablespoon of extra virgin olive oil. Cut the fish into pieces, add to the mixture and leave to marinate for at least 2 hours, or preferably overnight.

When you are ready to cook the dish, remove the fish pieces from the marinade and roll each piece in the cornflour. Heat 2 tablespoons of extra virgin olive oil in a large frying pan over medium heat, and fry the fish pieces until cooked through and golden brown.

To make the salad dressing, mix the soy sauce, vinegar, sugar, extra virgin olive oil and sesame oil until well combined. Season with salt and pepper.

To finish the salad, shred the cabbage, finely slice the carrot into thin sticks and slice the spring onions. Add the rice noodles and dressing and toss to combine. If using fried noodles, add them just before serving to ensure that they remain crisp. Serve the hot fish pieces with the salad.

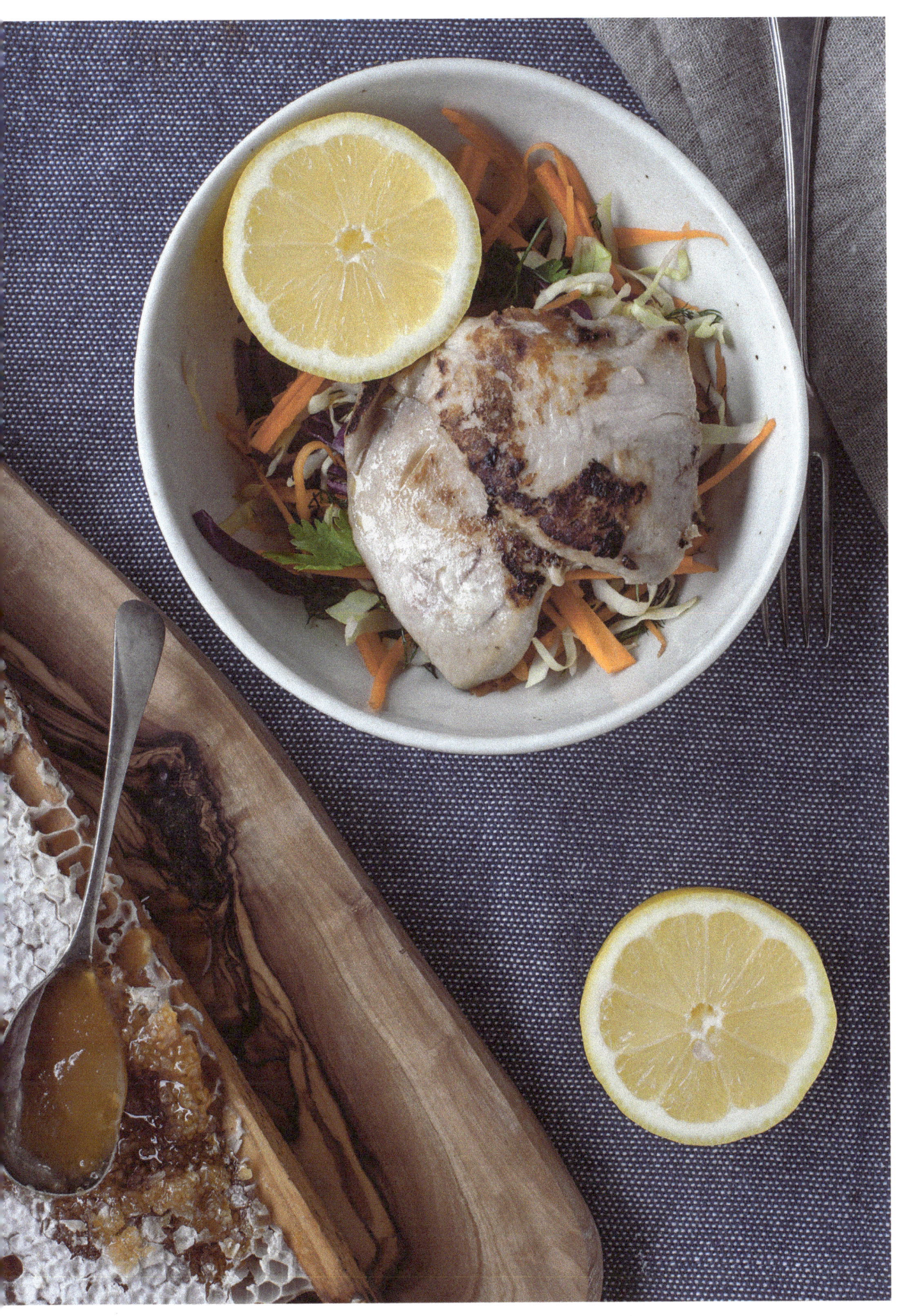

Fish and Potato Croquettes

SERVES 4 (MAKES 24)

These tasty croquettes are a number one hit with my kids, and are packed with vegetables. Kids will enjoy rolling them into a ball and coating them in the breadcrumbs. For an alternative option, replace the fish with beef mince. Whichever filling the kids choose, these croquettes are simply divine.

5 large Kennebec potatoes (or similar floury variety)

1 tablespoon butter

1 onion

1 carrot

1 clove garlic

extra virgin olive oil for pan frying

500 grams fish (steamed and flaked white fish or tinned fish)

1 zucchini

1 cup parmesan cheese

1 egg

salt and pepper

½ cup mixed fresh herbs

1 cup peas

1 ½ cups breadcrumbs

2-3 tablespoons extra virgin olive oil or extra virgin olive oil spray

Preheat oven to 180°C. Peel the potatoes and chop into 3cm dice. Place the potatoes in a saucepan of cold water and bring to the boil, reduce heat to medium and cook until tender. Drain the potatoes well, mash with the butter and set aside to cool.

Finely dice the onion, grate the carrot and crush the garlic. Heat the extra virgin olive oil in a heavy-based saucepan over medium heat, and saute the onion, carrot and garlic until soft. Add the fish and continue sautéing until cooked. Allow to cool slightly.

Grate the zucchini and add to the mashed potato along with the fish, parmesan cheese, egg, salt, pepper, herbs and peas. Use your hands to mix all the ingredients together until well combined. Shape tablespoons of mixture into small balls and flatten a little. Roll in breadcrumbs and arrange on a baking tray.

Drizzle with a little extra virgin olive oil or spray with extra virgin olive oil cooking spray and bake in the oven for 25 minutes or until golden. Turn them over then bake for another 10 minutes.

Serve warm with mild tomato chutney and a fresh crispy salad.

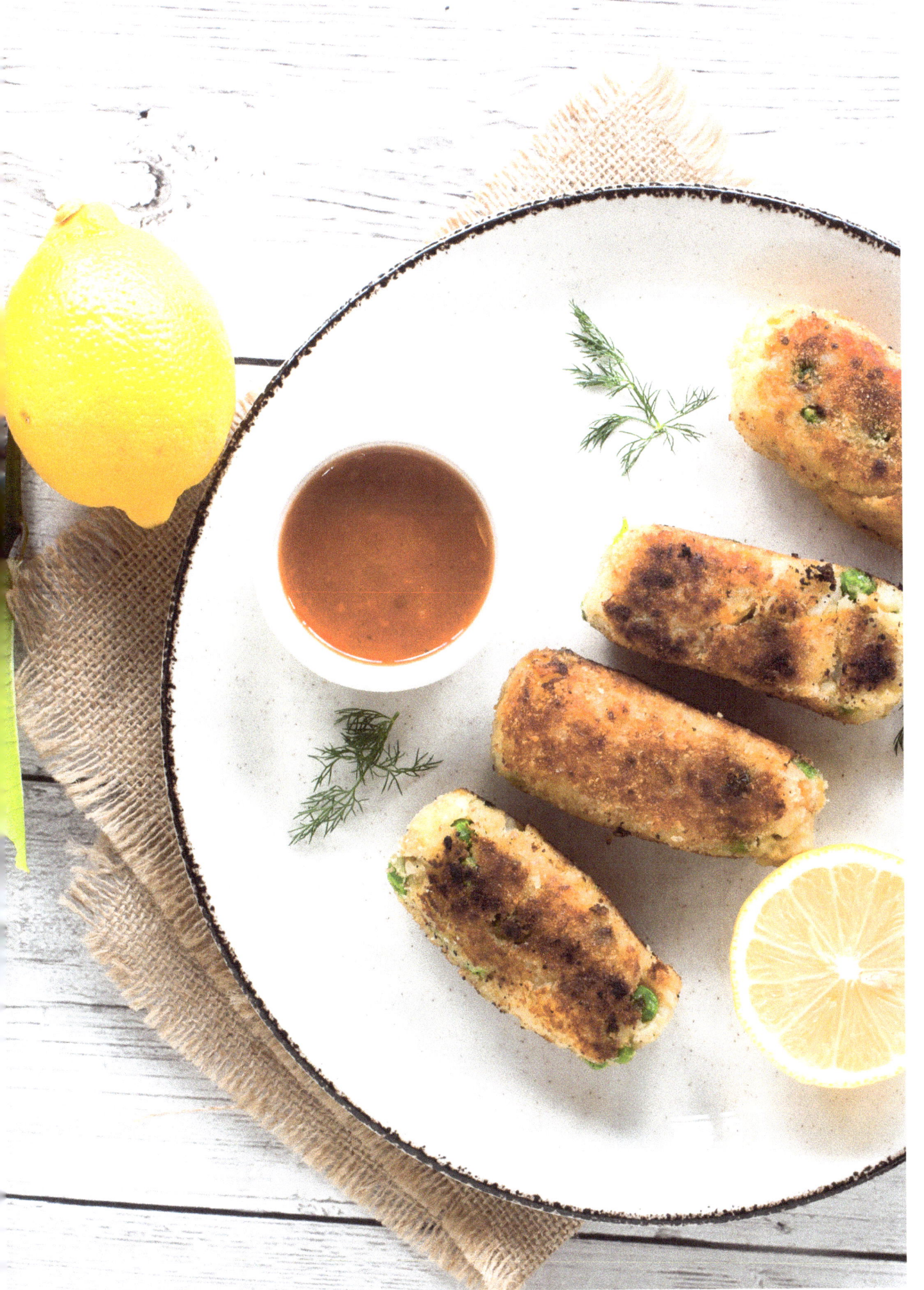

Spring Rolls

MAKES 20

A frozen fish such as albacore tuna is great to use in these spicy, deep fried spring rolls. Spring roll pastry is available from Asian grocers.

1 onion

1 clove garlic

1 large red chilli

1cm piece ginger

¼ small cabbage

2 carrots

300 grams fish

1 teaspoon sesame oil

1 tablespoon soy sauce

1 teaspoon fish sauce

1 cup cooked rice noodles

20 sheets spring roll pastry

1 egg for egg wash

extra virgin olive oil for deep or shallow frying

татов TO SERVE

dishes of sweet soy and sweet chili

To make the filling for the spring rolls, finely slice the onion, crush the peeled garlic, and finely chop the chilli and ginger. Finely slice the cabbage and coarsely grate the carrots. Chop the fish into 1cm dice. Heat the sesame oil in a large frying pan, or wok, over medium heat, and sauté the onion, garlic, chilli and ginger for a few minutes or until tender. Add the cabbage and carrot and continue to sauté for a few minutes until softened. Add the fish, soy and fish sauces and continue to sauté for a few minutes until the fish is almost cooked. Stir in the rice noodles. Leave to cool slightly before rolling.

Make the egg wash by whisking the egg in a small bowl.

To make the spring rolls, lay all the pastry sheets out on the bench. Working quickly to avoid the pastry drying out, put 2 large tablespoons of mixture 10cm from one corner of the pastry sheet, roll the top over and continue rolling tightly until half the sheet is used. Fold each side in and continue rolling, putting egg wash on the bottom corner to seal the pastry.

To deep fry the spring rolls, fill a deep saucepan or wok with extra virgin olive oil to a depth of at least 10cm, and heat the oil to 180°C. Check if the oil is hot enough by testing with a scrap of a spring roll wrapper – it should brown very quickly. Deep fry the rolls for about 3 minutes or until golden brown.

To shallow fry, heat a tablespoon of extra virgin olive oil in a heavy-based saucepan over medium heat. Fry the spring rolls for about 2 minutes on each side or until golden and crispy.

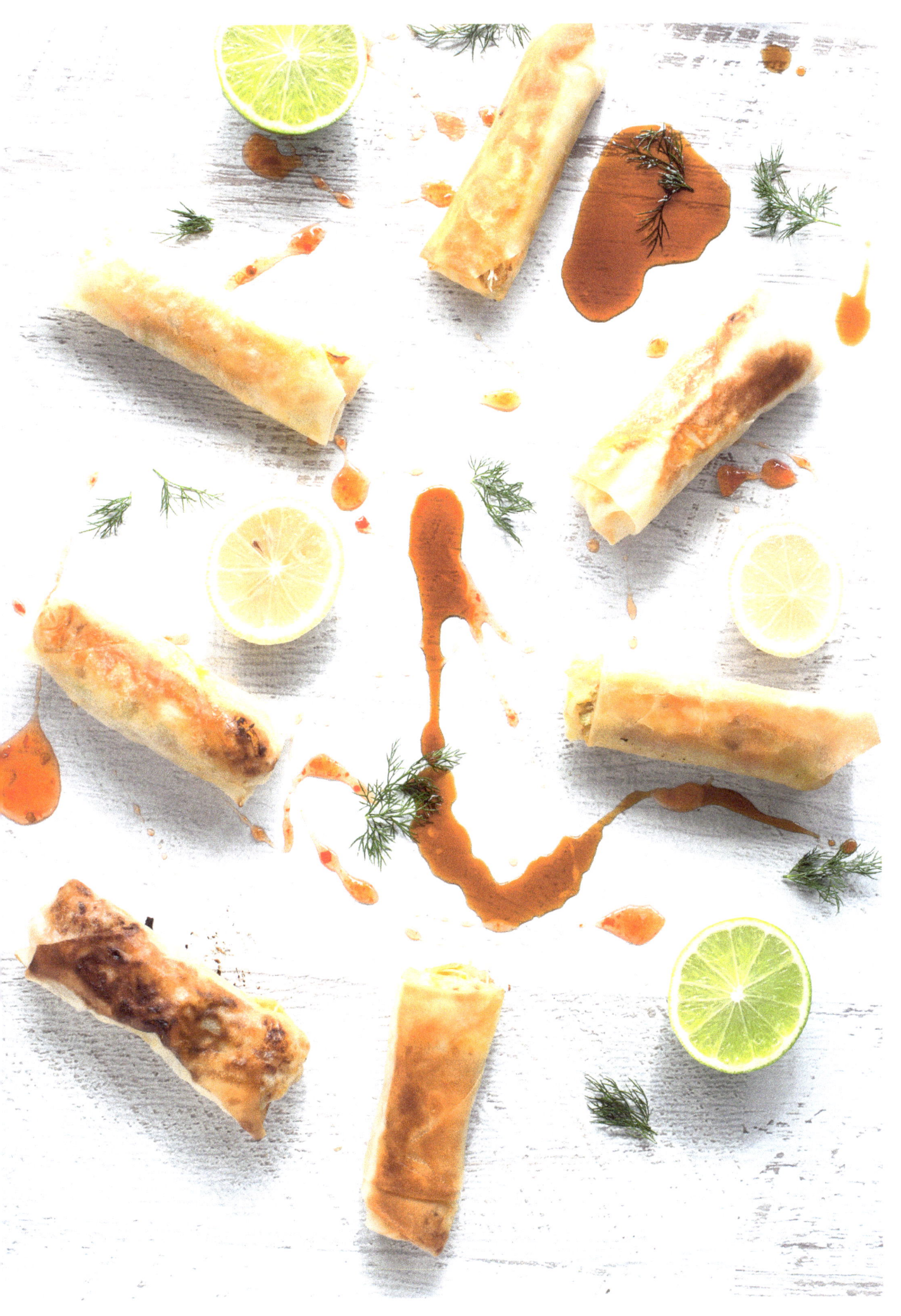

Beer Battered Fish

SERVES 4

A traditional favourite, and for good reason! We like this best served with homemade chips, tartare sauce and crisp green salad. If you don't have a deep fryer, use a deep saucepan of extra virgin olive oil to cook the fish, and take care to avoid any hot splatters.

extra virgin olive oil for deep-frying

1 ½ cups self-raising flour

1 tablespoon vinegar

1 can (375ml) beer

800 grams fish fillets

3 tablespoons plain flour

Heat your deep fryer, or saucepan of extra virgin olive oil to 180°C. If you are using a saucepan of oil, fill to a depth of at least 10cm and use a cooking thermometer to test the temperature.

To make the batter, whisk together the self-raising flour, vinegar and beer in a large bowl.

Cut the fish fillets into pieces, preferably no more than 15 mm thick. Sprinkle the plain flour onto a plate. Press both sides of the fish fillets into the flour and shake off excess. Dunk the fillets in the batter, ensuring they are fully coated.

Carefully lower the fish fillets into the hot oil and cook for 5 minutes or until golden brown and cooked through.

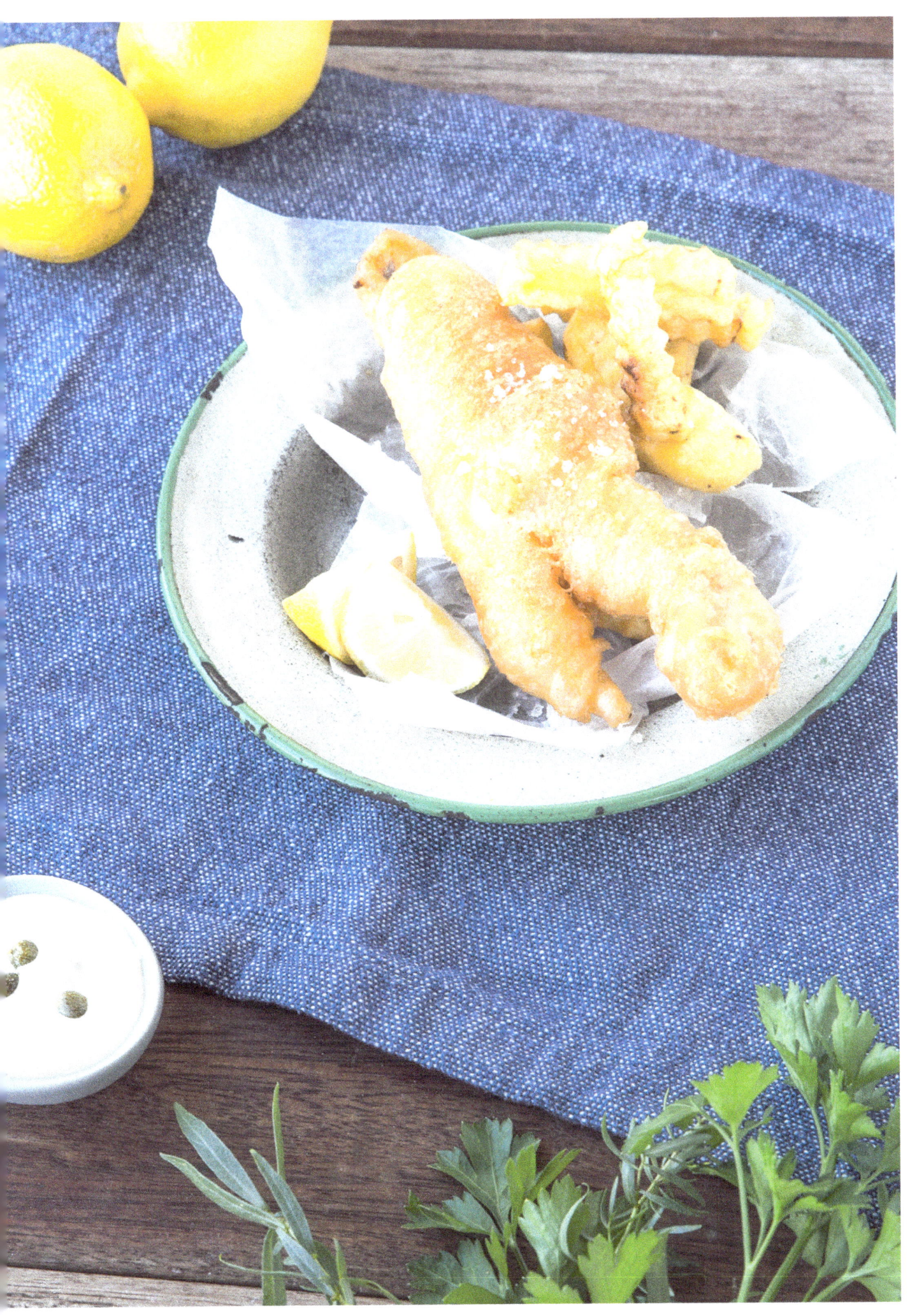

Whole Baked Fish with Feta, Roast Bintje Potatoes, Spinach and Skordallia

SERVES 4

LEMON AND OREGANO DRESSING
2 tablespoons oregano
1 tablespoon extra virgin olive oil
1 tablespoon lemon juice

POTATOES
600 grams baby Bintje potatoes
2 tablespoons extra virgin olive oil
3 cloves garlic
300 grams spinach leaves
150 grams feta cheese

SKORDALLIA
250 grams potatoes
1 egg
50ml white wine vinegar
salt and pepper
3 cloves garlic
1 tablespoon lemon juice
100ml extra virgin olive oil

BAKED FISH
whole white fish approximately 1kg
plain flour
extra virgin olive oil for pan-frying

Preheat the oven to 180°C.

To make the dressing, finely chop the oregano and mix with the extra virgin olive oil and lemon juice.

Wash the potatoes and chop into 2 cm dice. Add the extra virgin olive oil, garlic and potatoes to a baking tray and roast for about 25 minutes, or until cooked through and crispy. Toss the spinach and feta through the hot potatoes just before serving.

To make the skordallia, peel and dice the remaining potatoes. Put potatoes into a large saucepan, cover with water, bring to the boil and cook for 15-20 minutes or until cooked through. Drain well and set aside to cool slightly. Using a food processor, blend the potatoes with the egg, vinegar, a pinch of salt and pepper, garlic and lemon juice until well combined and smooth. While still blending, add the extra virgin olive oil in a slow drizzle until the potato mix is thick and creamy.

To cook the fish, heat the extra virgin olive oil in an ovenproof pan over medium heat. Coat the fish in flour and cook for a few minutes on each side, until the skin is crispy and golden brown. Transfer the pan to the oven to finish cooking the fish – this will take approximately 10 minutes, depending on the size of the fish. Drizzle the hot fish with the lemon and oregano dressing and serve with the warm potato salad and skordallia.

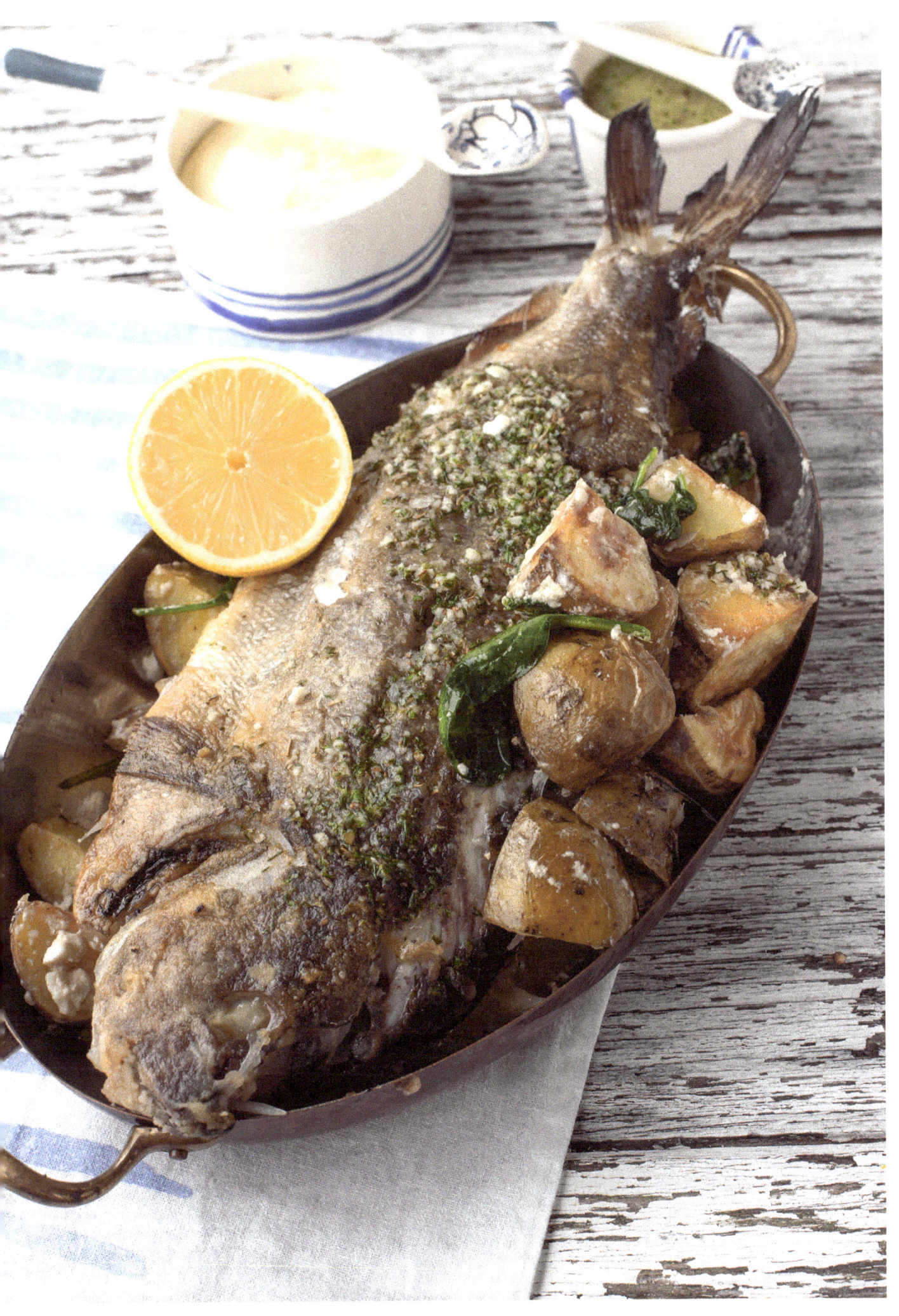

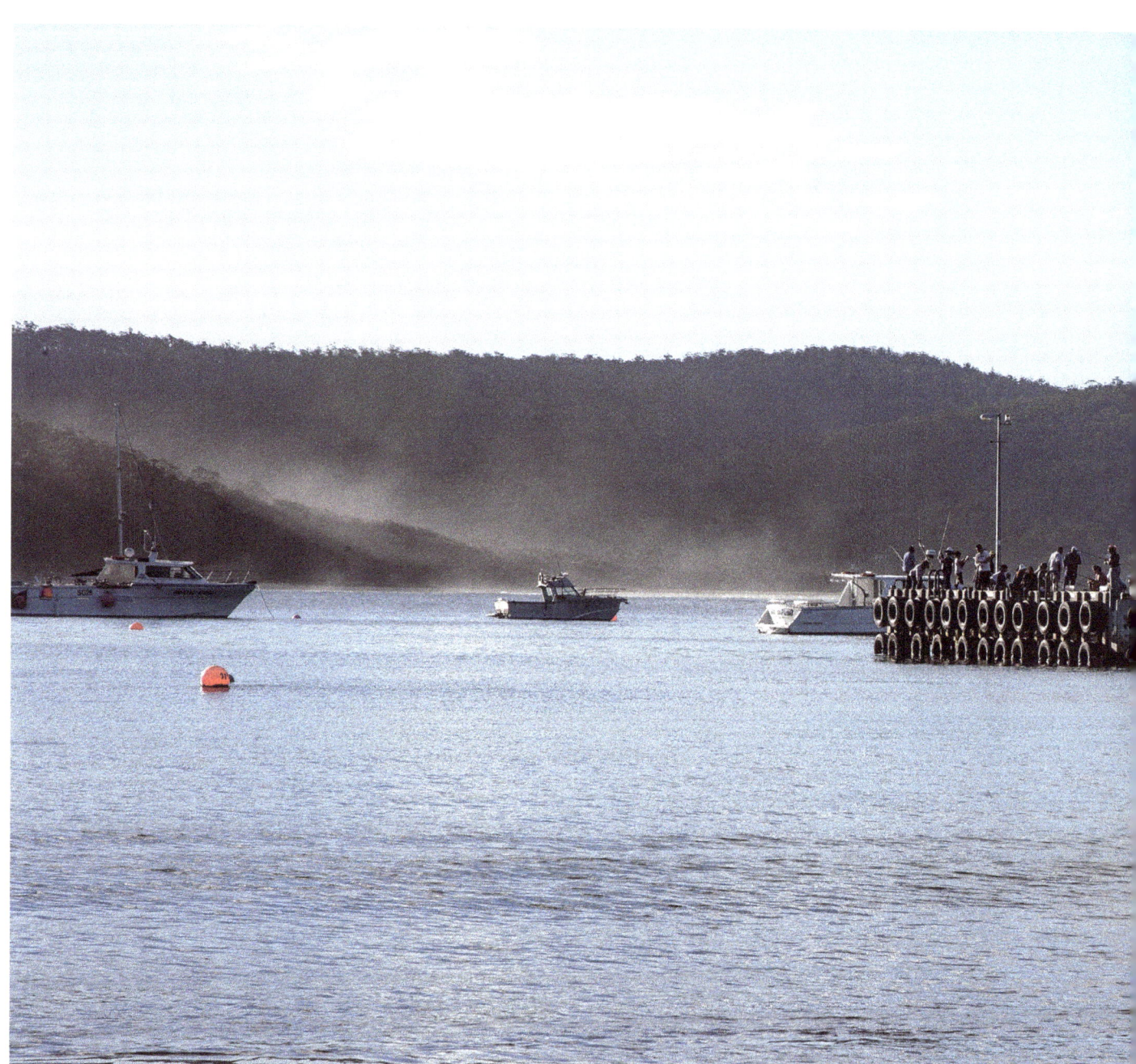

Cephalopods

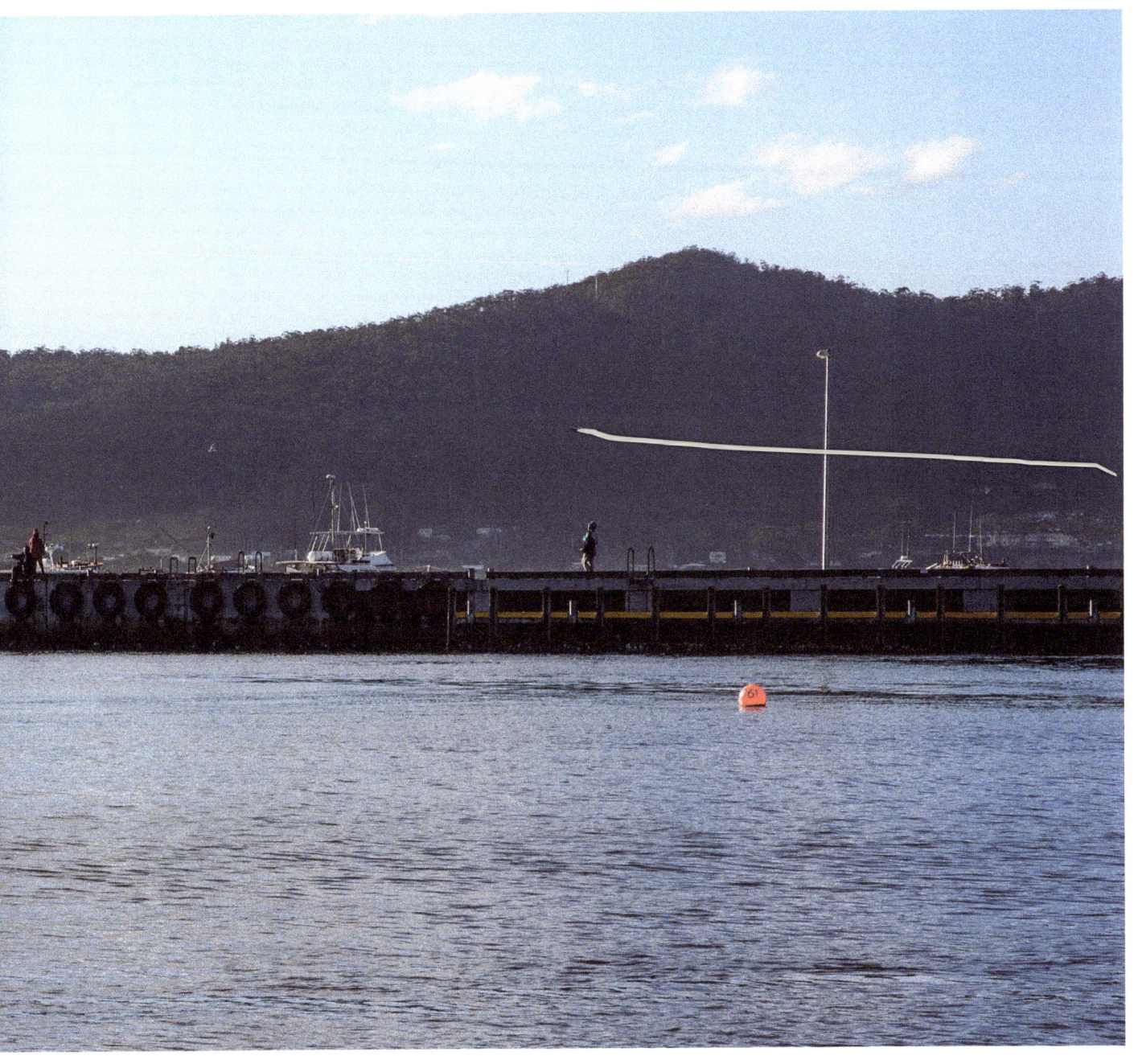

Salt and Sichuan Peppered Squid with Lemon Aioli

SERVES 4-6

Fishing for squid is great fun, especially with kids! We love fishing for them off the jetty at Eaglehawk Neck and cheer each other on as the squid are hooked and pulled up one by one. If you do catch the squid yourself, don't forget to prepare legs as well as the body – they are full of flavor even if they can be a bit chewy, and they are my favourite part! If you haven't prepared a squid before it is not difficult to do, just be careful not to pop the ink sac to avoid a mess.

LEMON AIOLI

2 egg yolks

1 egg

1 tablespoon white vinegar

1 lemon, juice and zest

1 clove garlic

salt and pepper

200ml extra virgin olive oil

SALT AND SICHUAN PEPPERED SQUID

4 whole fresh squid (or calamari), tubes and legs

2 cups plain flour

1 tablespoon salt

1 tablespoon cracked Sichuan peppercorns

extra virgin olive oil for frying

To make the aioli, use a blender or food processor to combine the egg yolks, whole egg, vinegar, lemon juice and zest, crushed garlic and a pinch of salt and pepper. While still blending, slowly add the extra virgin olive oil in a steady drizzle to create a thick and creamy emulsion.

To clean the squid, remove the tube from the legs. Cut each leg off and discard innards. Turn the squid tube inside out and remove the spine by pulling out the cartilage. Remove the skin from the squid tube. Cut the squid into rings about 1cm thick. Put flour, salt and pepper into a plastic bag and shake to combine, then add the squid rings and whole legs. Shake the bag well to coat all of the tubes and legs with the flour mixture.

To deep fry, heat extra virgin olive oil to about 170°C and cook the squid in batches for about 4 minutes, or until golden brown. To shallow fry, heat a few tablespoons of oil over medium heat and fry squid for 2-3 minutes on each side or until cooked through.

Drain on paper towel to remove excess oil and serve immediately with the lemon aioli and a crisp salad.

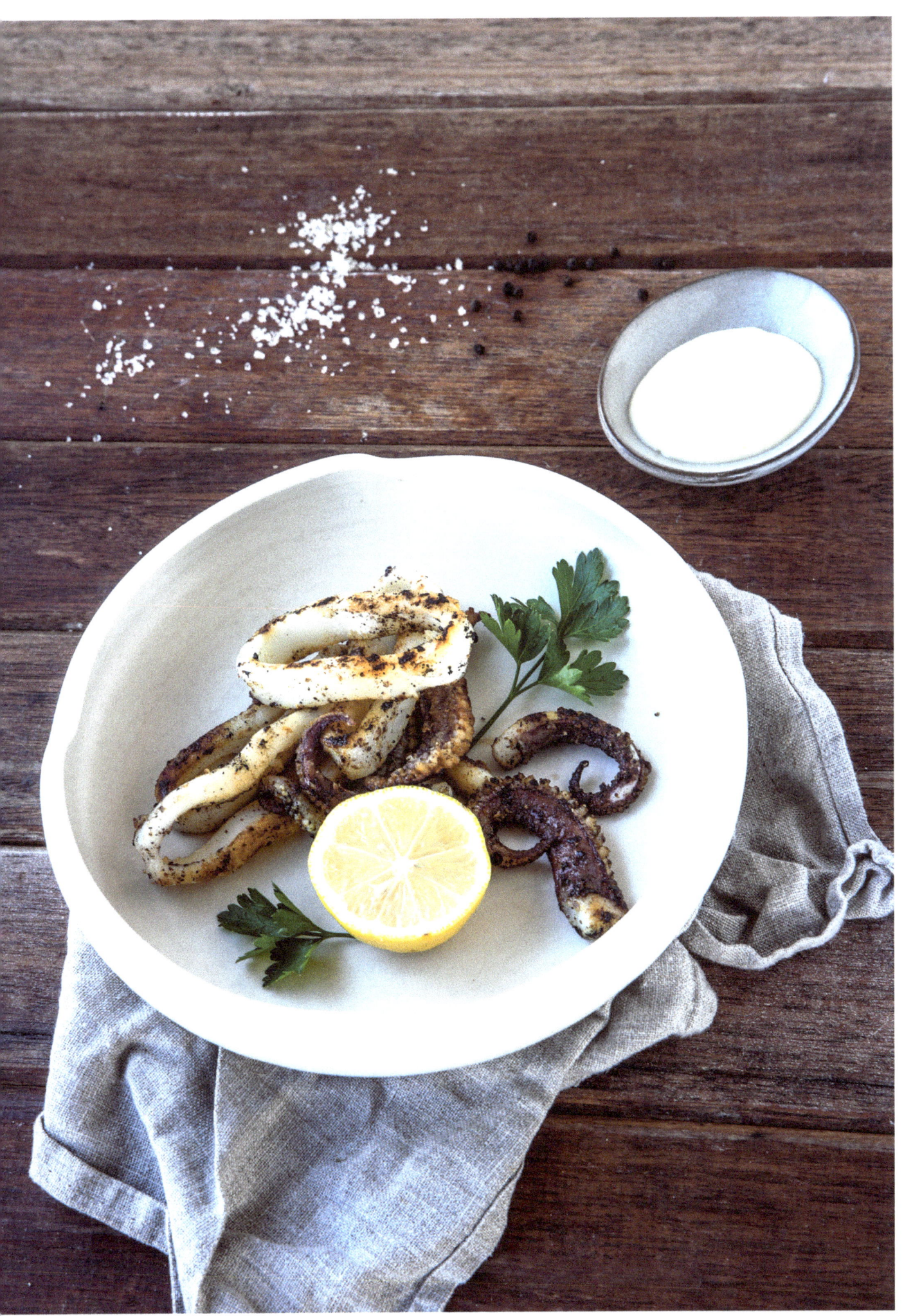

Stuffed Squid with Red Pepper Sauce

SERVES 4

The stuffing for the squid and the red pepper sauce can both be prepared in advance and refrigerated until needed. This recipe is a great alternative method of cooking squid and is a fabulous dinner party dish.

RED PEPPER SAUCE

3 red capsicums

1 tablespoon extra virgin olive oil

2 cloves garlic

1 small onion

1 cup cream

STUFFED SQUID

1 small onion

1 clove garlic

⅔ cup Arborio or short grain rice

2 ½ cups fish stock

1 cup spinach

100 grams feta cheese

50 grams parmesan

4 large squid tubes

2 tablespoons extra virgin olive oil

TO BAKE

extra virgin olive oil

3 cloves of garlic

1 lemon

To make the sauce, preheat the oven to 180°C, rub the capsicums with a small amount of extra virgin olive oil and roast in the oven for 10 minutes - or until the capsicums have softened and the skin is blackened. Remove capsicums from the oven, place in a bowl and cover with plastic wrap, this will make the capsicums easier to peel. Once the capsicums have cooled enough to handle, peel off the skins. Remove and discard the seeds. Slice the capsicum into strips.

Peel and finely dice the onion and garlic. Using a heavy-based saucepan, heat the remaining oil over medium heat and sauté the onion and garlic. Add the sliced capsicum and cream and bring to the boil. Reduce heat and simmer for 10 minutes or until all of the vegetables are softened. Using a stick blender, blend until smooth. Set aside until required.

To make the stuffed squid, finely dice the onion and crush the garlic. Heat the extra virgin olive oil in a heavy-based saucepan over medium heat, and sauté the onion and garlic until softened. Add the rice and cook, stirring for one minute. Add the stock, bring to a simmer and continue to simmer whilst stirring, until the rice is cooked. This will take approximately 25 minutes. Set aside to cool. Chop the spinach, crumble the feta and grate the parmesan cheese. Once the mixture has cooled, mix the spinach and cheeses into the rice.

To stuff the squid, use a toothpick or skewer to firmly close one end of the squid tube. Fill the tube with the stuffing mix and then use a toothpick or skewer to close the other end of the squid tube.

Place the squid tubes in a baking dish and rub with extra virgin olive oil add the roughly chopped up garlic and lemon to the baking dish. Bake in the oven for approximately 25 minutes, or until the squid is cooked and the filling is heated through.

To serve, carefully slice the squid tubes and serve with the warm red pepper sauce.

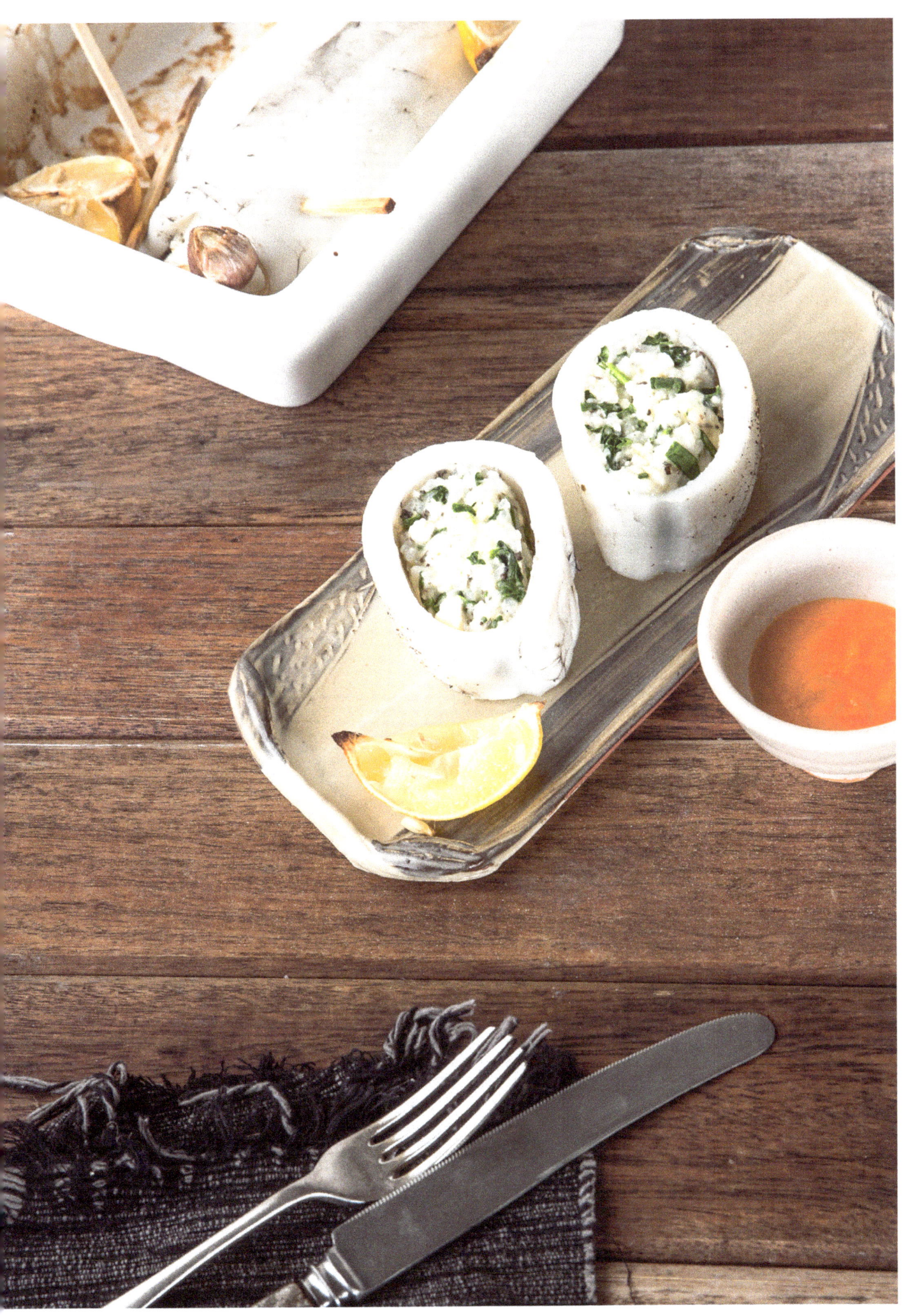

Barbequed Octopus with Pea, Cabbage and Feta Salad

SERVES 4

This salad is a fabulous accompaniment to all types of seafood; the peas and fresh herbs give it a wonderful fresh flavour. Eaglehawk Neck is well known for being a great place to catch octopus, and we are lucky enough to be able to buy freshly caught octopus from our local farmers market. We also sometimes find octopus that have crawled into our craypots when we set them overnight! You could try sourcing octopus from your local fish market or asking your fishmonger, or tell your cray-fishing friends to keep their eyes out for any stowaways! If you can only get hold of frozen octopus, that's OK! Octopus is actually more tender when it has been frozen first and then defrosted.

BBQ OCTOPUS

800 grams octopus legs

2 cloves garlic

1 tablespoon oregano

extra virgin olive oil

1 teaspoon cracked black pepper

SALAD

2 cups green peas fresh or frozen

⅛ cabbage

1 small bunch chives

100 grams feta

salt and pepper

2 lemons

1 clove garlic

2 tablespoons oregano

2 tablespoons parsley

½ tablespoon mint

1 tablespoons extra virgin olive oil

If you have caught the octopus yourself, you will need to clean the legs. Sprinkle salt on your fingers to help grip the octopus and pull all of the skin off the legs. Discard the skin. Rinse the legs and set aside.

To make the marinade for the octopus, crush the garlic, finely chop the oregano and mix with the extra virgin olive oil. Pour over the octopus legs. Grind over the black pepper and set aside to marinate for at least 3 hours.

To make the salad, bring a small saucepan of water to the boil and cook the peas for one minute. Drain and set aside to cool. Finely slice the cabbage and chop the chives. Chop the feta into ½ cm pieces and mix with the cabbage, peas and chives. To make the dressing, juice the lemon, crush the garlic and mix with the chopped oregano, parsley, mint and extra virgin olive oil. Pour the dressing over the salad and toss lightly to combine.

To cook the octopus, heat the flat grill of the barbeque (or frying pan) to a very high heat. Grill the octopus legs for about 8 minutes, turning regularly. Cooking time will depend on the thickness of the legs. The octopus is cooked though when it is firm to the touch and white all the way through. Serve the octopus immediately, with the salad on the side.

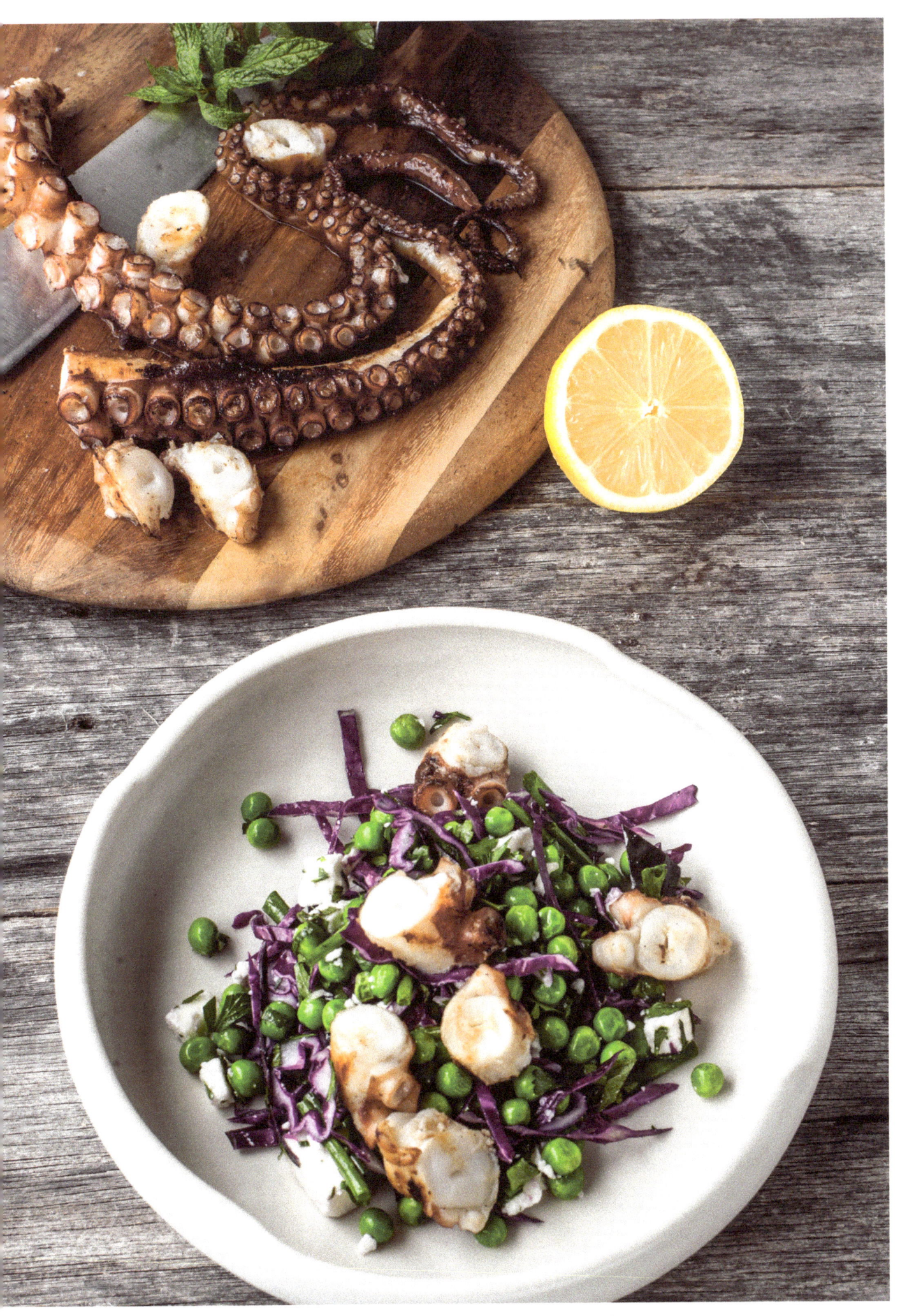

Barbequed Octopus with Feta Risotto Balls and Lemon Aioli

SERVES 4

Cooking freshly caught octopus on the barbeque is a wonderful summer treat – the smoky, chargrilled flavour is delicious.

BARBEQUED OCTOPUS

800 grams octopus legs

2 cloves garlic

1 tablespoon fresh oregano

extra virgin olive oil

1 teaspoon cracked pepper

RISOTTO BALLS

2 cups chicken stock

1 medium onion

⅔ cup Arborio rice

1 tablespoon extra virgin olive oil

100 grams feta cheese

1 tablespoon oregano

¼ teaspoon salt

¼ teaspoon pepper

1 egg

1 cup milk

1 cup flour

1 cup bread crumbs

LEMON AIOLI

2 egg yolks

1 egg

1 tablespoon white vinegar

1 lemon, juice and zest

1 clove garlic

salt and pepper

200ml extra virgin olive oil

extra virgin olive oil for deep-frying

To prepare the octopus, pull off all of the skin and discard. To remove the skin use some salt on your fingers for grip and pull it off. Don't be too fussy around the tentacles.

To make the marinade, crush the garlic, chop the oregano and combine with the extra virgin olive oil and pepper. Marinate the octopus in this mixture for a few hours, or overnight if possible.

To make the risotto balls, bring the stock to the boil in a saucepan. In a separate heavy-based saucepan, heat the extra virgin olive oil over medium heat and sauté the finely diced onion until translucent. Add the rice and cook stirring for one minute. Add the stock one ladle at a time and continue stirring until mostly absorbed. Continue with this process until the rice is cooked, or about 20 minutes. Remove from the heat and set aside to cool. Crumble the feta cheese, chop the oregano and stir through the risotto along with the salt and pepper. Roll the risotto into balls about the size of a 20 cent piece, place on a tray lined with baking paper and refrigerate for an hour, or until firm.

To prepare the risotto balls, crack the egg into a bowl and whisk lightly with the milk. Place the flour and breadcrumbs in two separate bowls. Remove risotto balls from refrigerator. Roll each ball in the flour, shake off excess, dip the ball into the egg mixture, shake off excess and then roll in breadcrumbs. Repeat with all of the balls. Place onto a baking tray and refrigerate until ready to use.

To cook the octopus, heat the flat grill of the BBQ (or a frying pan) over very high heat. Cook the marinated octopus legs for about 8 minutes (depending on the thickness of the legs) turning regularly. The octopus is cooked when it is firm to the touch and white all the way through.

To make the aioli, use a blender or food processor to combine the egg yolks, whole egg, vinegar, lemon juice and zest, crushed garlic and a pinch of salt and pepper. While still blending, slowly add the oil in a steady drizzle to create a thick and creamy emulsion.

To cook the risotto balls, heat a deep fryer filled with oil or fill a saucepan with oil to at least 6cm deep and heat until it reaches 170°C. Cook the balls in small batches for about 4 minutes or until golden brown. Alternatively, use a deep fryer if you wish. Drain on paper towel and serve immediately with the octopus and aioli.

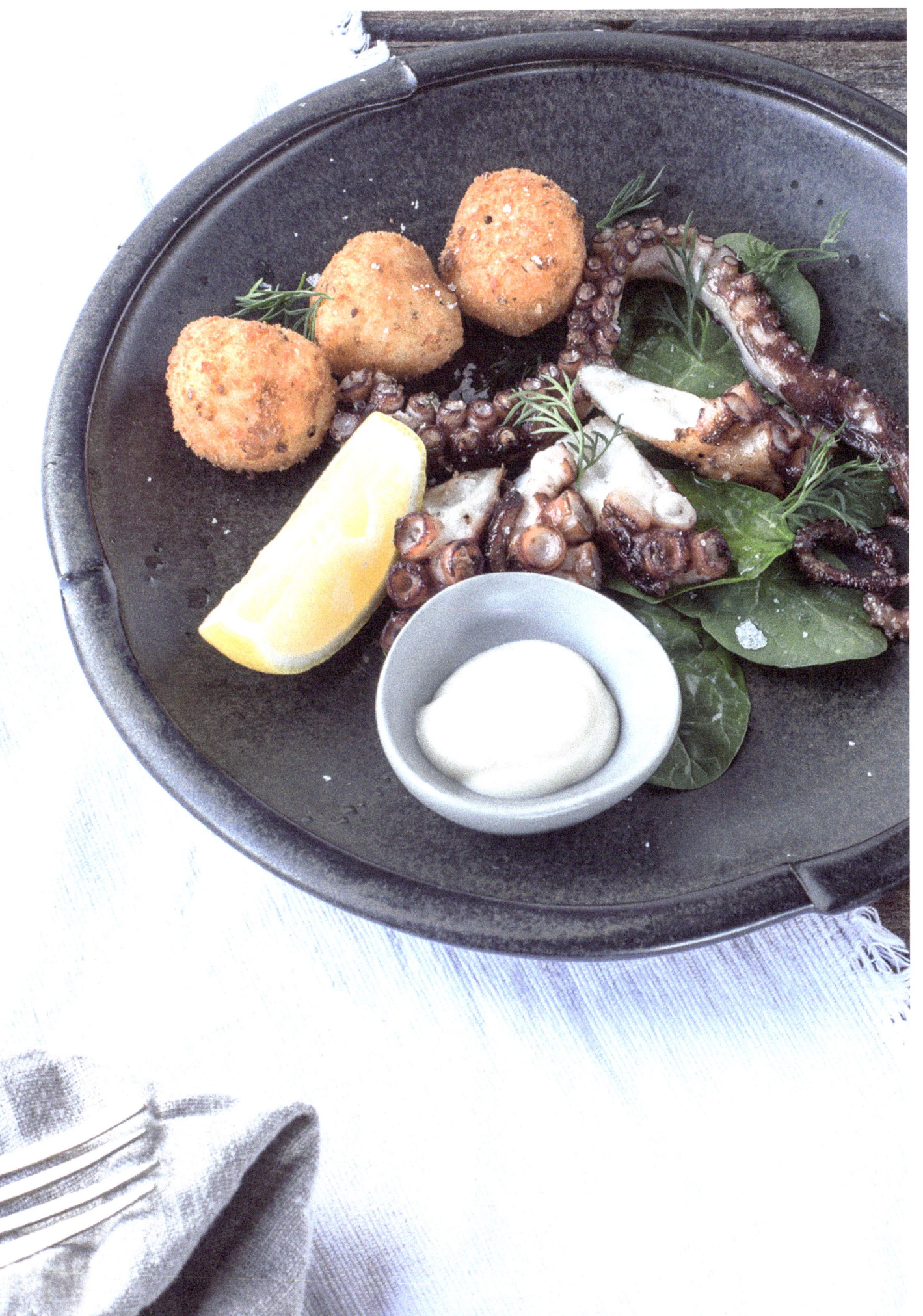

Squid Spaghetti with Lemon and Garlic

SERVES 4

If you like eating squid legs, you can include them in this recipe along with the tubes. I have used a food processor to make the pasta dough here, as it is a very quick and easy method - however if you prefer to make it by hand the method is on page 30.

SPAGHETTI

2 cups plain flour

1 tablespoon extra virgin olive oil

2 eggs

additional flour for dusting

SQUID

4 squid tubes

4 cloves garlic

2 medium brown onions

4 tablespoons tarragon

3 lemons

1 tablespoon extra virgin olive oil

50 grams butter

salt and pepper

100 grams parmesan cheese

Use a food processor to make the pasta dough. Place the flour in the food processor. Turn on the processor and with the motor running, add the oil and the eggs. Continue blending until the mixture comes together to form a firm dough. If the mixture seems too wet or sticky to handle, knead in a little more flour by hand on a floured bench.

To roll the pasta, divide the dough into 4 portions. Using a pasta machine set at number 1 (or at the widest setting) feed each portion of the dough through the machine. Repeat this process with each portion of pasta on each setting, until you reach setting number 6, (or the highest setting on your machine) the pasta should be silky smooth and slightly elastic. Cut the pasta into spaghetti strips using the appropriate cutter on the pasta machine. Dust the bench with flour and carefully lay the lengths of dough aside until needed.

To cook the spaghetti, bring a large saucepan of salted water to the boil and cook the spaghetti for 4 minutes. Alternatively the pasta can be cooked in advance, even the day before it is required. To do so, simply cook the spaghetti as above, cool and roll in a little extra virgin olive oil and refrigerate until required. Reheat the spaghetti in the sauce when you are ready to serve the dish.

To cook the squid, slice the squid into strips about 5mm wide. If the legs are large they can be cut in half. Crush the garlic, finely slice the onion and finely chop the tarragon. Juice the lemons. Heat a large heavy-based pan over medium heat, add the oil and sauté the onion, garlic and squid for about 5 minutes, or until the squid is cooked and the onion is soft. Avoid overcooking, as this will make the squid tough. Add the butter and lemon juice to the pan, and season well with salt and pepper. Toss the spaghetti through the hot sauce, add the tarragon and serve immediately with the shaved parmesan cheese.

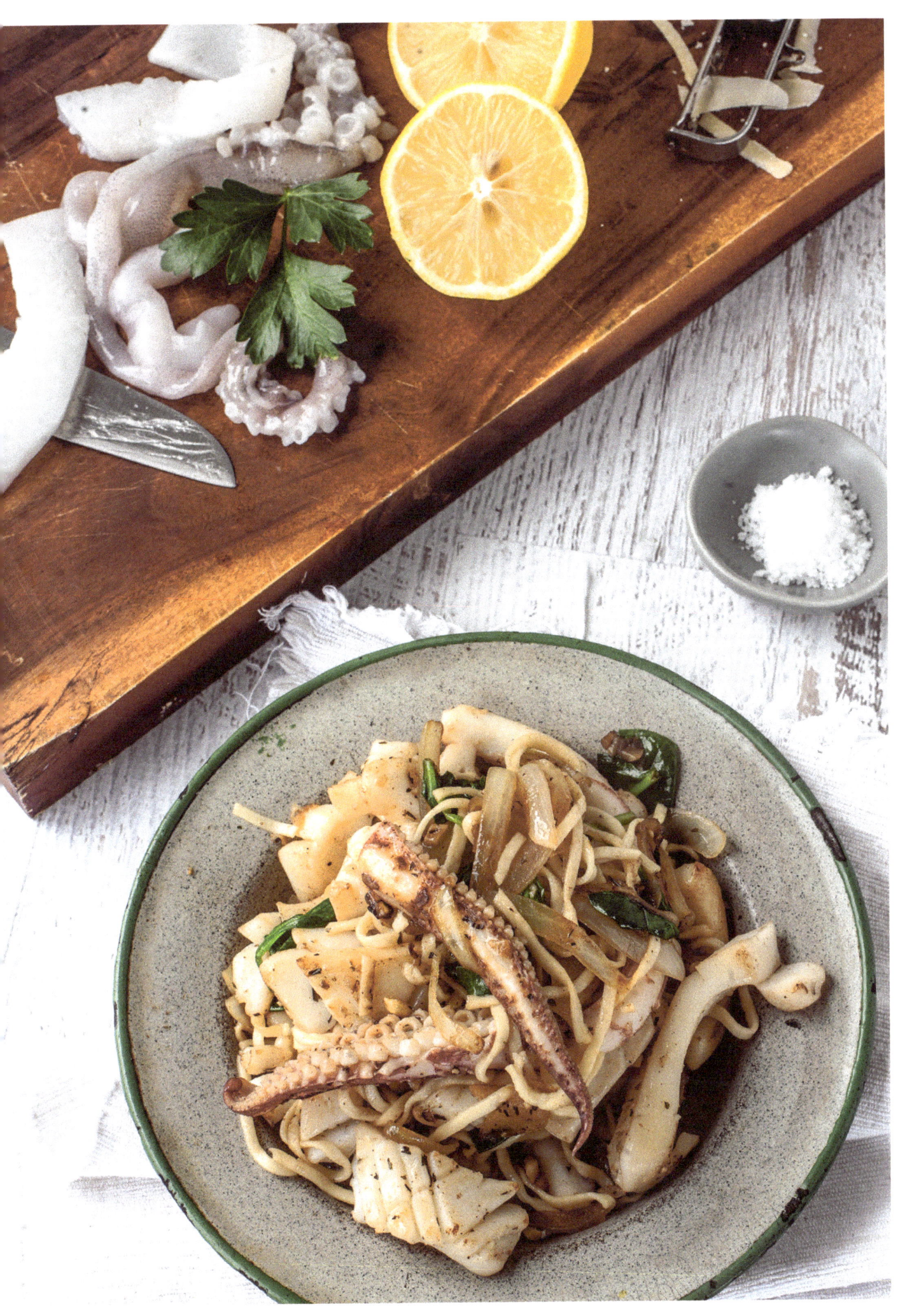

Pickled Octopus with a Greek Style Salad

SERVES 4

If you're lucky enough to be able to set your own cray pots, or if you live in a popular fishing area, you may have noticed that octopus turn up in the cray pots fairly regularly. Lots of people are not really sure what to do with them, but this method of pickling is delicious, easy, and a much better option that using the octopus for bait! This is the pickling method of that I learnt when I worked in a Greek restaurant and it results in amazingly tender octopus. You can store the pickled octopus in extra virgin olive oil for a few weeks. It is lovely served with salads, or antipasto, or it can be a meal on it's own. To clean the octopus, refer to the notes on page 98.

PICKLED OCTOPUS

1 onion

1 teaspoon garlic

1 large chilli

1 teaspoon oregano

1 lemon diced

1 kilogram octopus, cleaned and cut into 10cm pieces

½ teaspoon salt

½ teaspoon pepper

1 litre extra virgin olive oil (approximately)

SALAD DRESSING

1 tablespoon oregano

1 clove garlic

100ml extra virgin olive oil

50ml red wine vinegar

pinch of salt and pepper

SALAD

2 tomatoes

1 cucumber

1 Spanish onion

100 grams feta cheese

100 grams olives

To pickle the octopus, finely chop the onion, garlic, chilli and oregano. Using a heavy-based saucepan, heat 1 teaspoon of the extra virgin olive oil over medium heat and sauté the onion, garlic, chilli and oregano for a few minutes, or until the onions have softened. Add the octopus, and stir and fry until all of the surfaces are sealed. Add the lemon, season with salt and pepper, reduce the heat and cook gently for 5 minutes or until a lot of the liquid has come out of the octopus.

Top with enough oil to completely cover the octopus. Reduce heat to low and cook for 40 minutes, simmering gently. Cut a piece of octopus to test if it is cooked – it should be soft, opaque and cooked through. Remove the saucepan from the heat, cover with a lid and set aside to tenderise and cool for at least 3 hours. Once cooled, place in the refrigerator.

To make the salad dressing, chop the oregano, crush the garlic and mix with the oil, vinegar, salt and pepper. Slice the tomatoes, cucumber and onion, crumble the feta cheese and combine with the olives. To serve, assemble the salad and octopus on a plate or large platter and drizzle over the dressing.

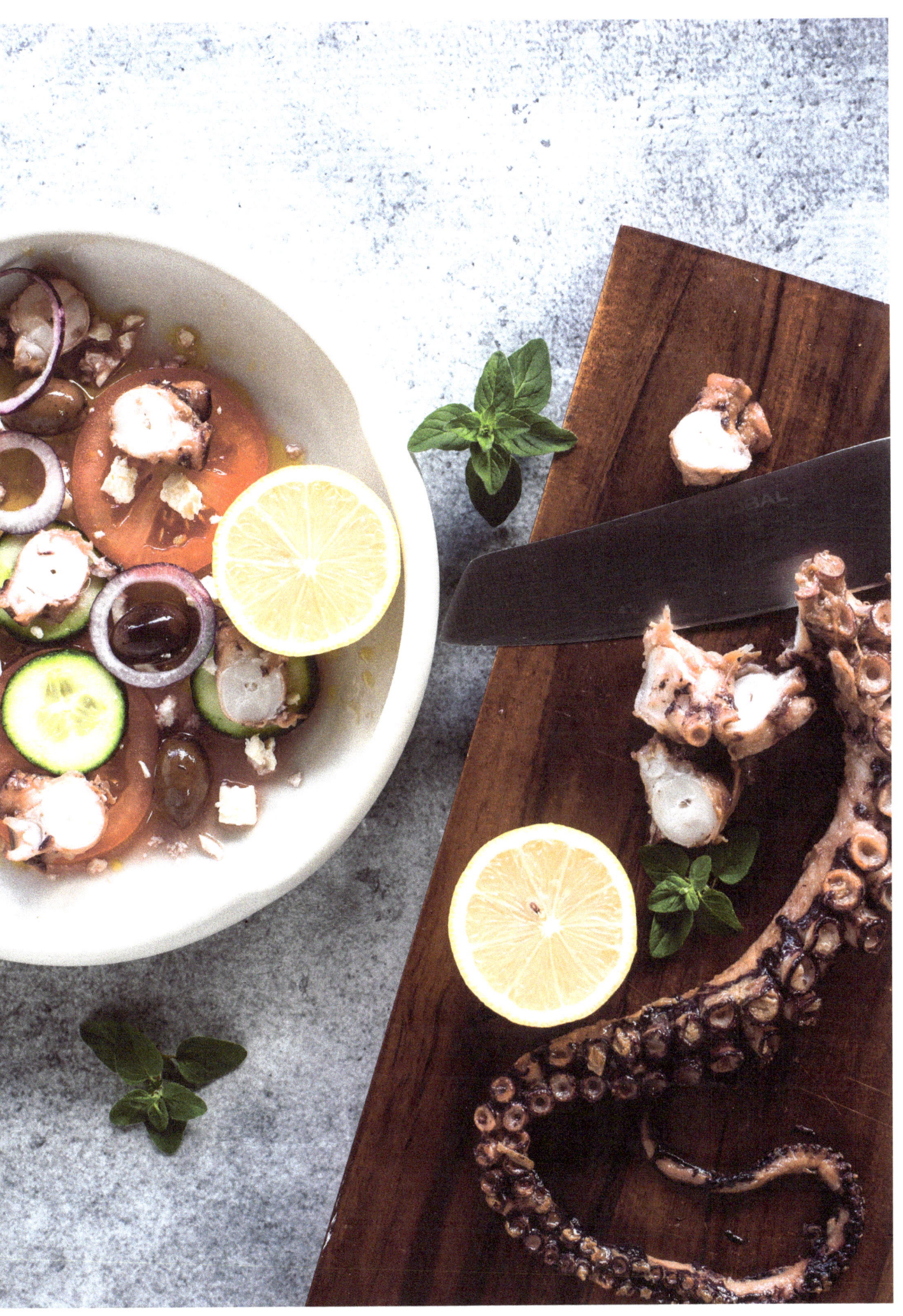

Grilled Octopus with Spinach and Cheese Pie

SERVES 4-6

SPINACH AND CHEESE PIE

1 onion

1 clove garlic

1 tablespoon extra virgin olive oil

200 grams spinach leaves

150 grams feta cheese

150 grams ricotta cheese

80 grams parmesan cheese

salt and pepper

50 grams butter

1 packet filo pastry

GRILLED OCTOPUS

2 cloves garlic

1 tablespoon fresh oregano

extra virgin olive oil

1 teaspoon cracked pepper

800 grams octopus legs

Pre-heat the oven to 180°C.

To make the pie, finely chop the onion and garlic. Heat the extra virgin olive oil in a heavy-based saucepan over medium heat and sauté the onion and garlic until softened. Add the spinach and continue to sauté until just cooked. Drain any liquid from the saucepan and set aside to cool. Grate the parmesan cheese, and crumble the feta. Stir the ricotta, parmesan and feta cheeses through the spinach mix and season with salt and pepper. Melt the butter and set aside. Carefully unwrap the filo pastry and separate into 4 equal portions. Use ¼ of the pastry sheets to line the bottom of a medium-sized baking tray, brushing each sheet with butter before layering with the next. Top with ⅓ of the spinach mix. Repeat the layering process in the same manner, ensuring that the top layer is pastry. Brush the top with melted butter and bake for 15-20 minutes or until the pastry is golden brown.

To marinate the octopus, crush the garlic, finely chop the oregano and combine with the extra virgin olive oil and cracked pepper. Pour over the octopus legs and set aside to marinate for at least one hour.

To cook the octopus, heat the grill plate of a barbeque, or a frying pan on the stove, over very high heat. Cook the octopus legs for approximately 8 minutes, turning regularly. The legs may need more or less cooking time depending on their thickness. The legs will be cooked when white and opaque all the way through.

Serve the octopus legs with a slice of spinach and cheese pie.

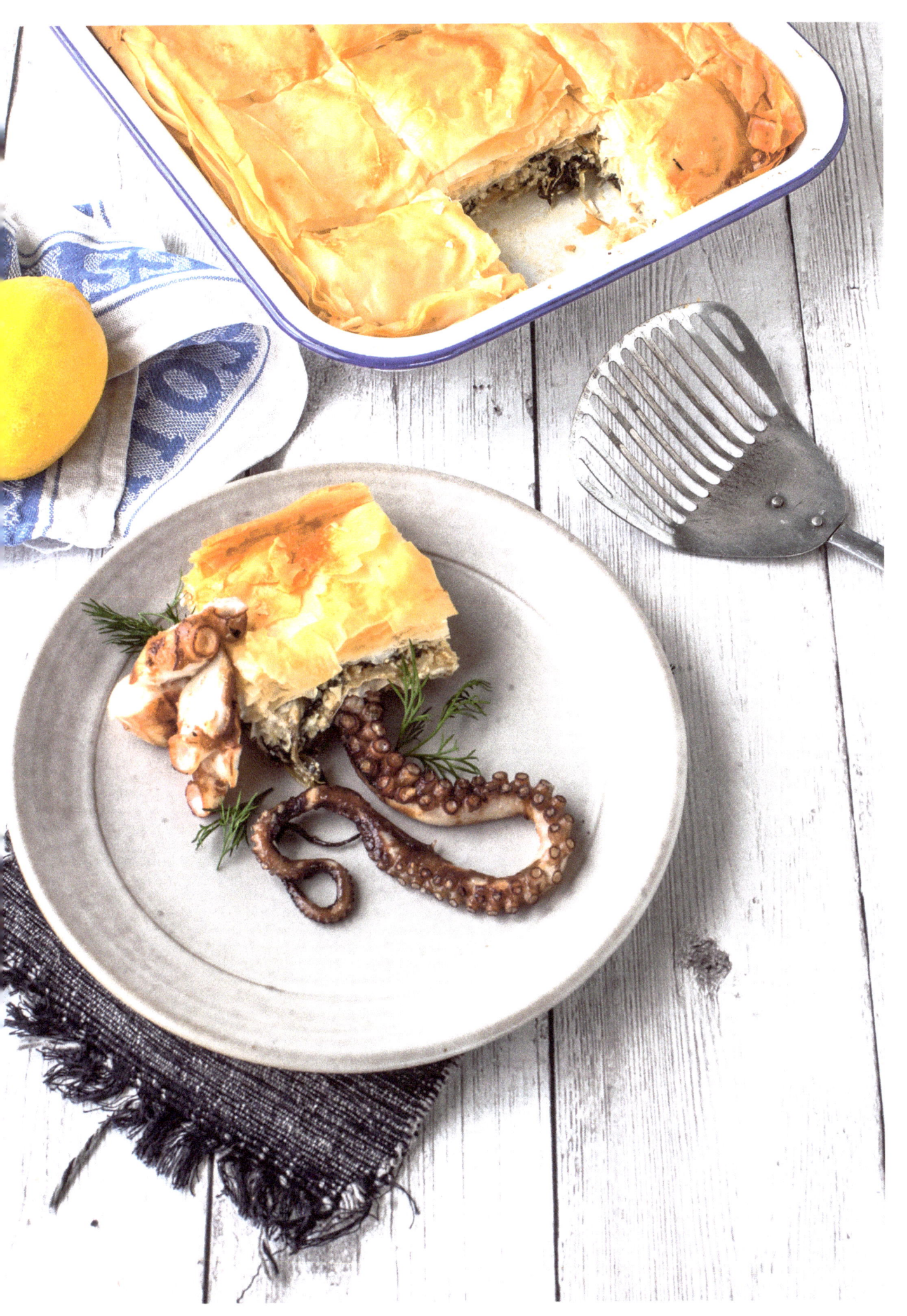

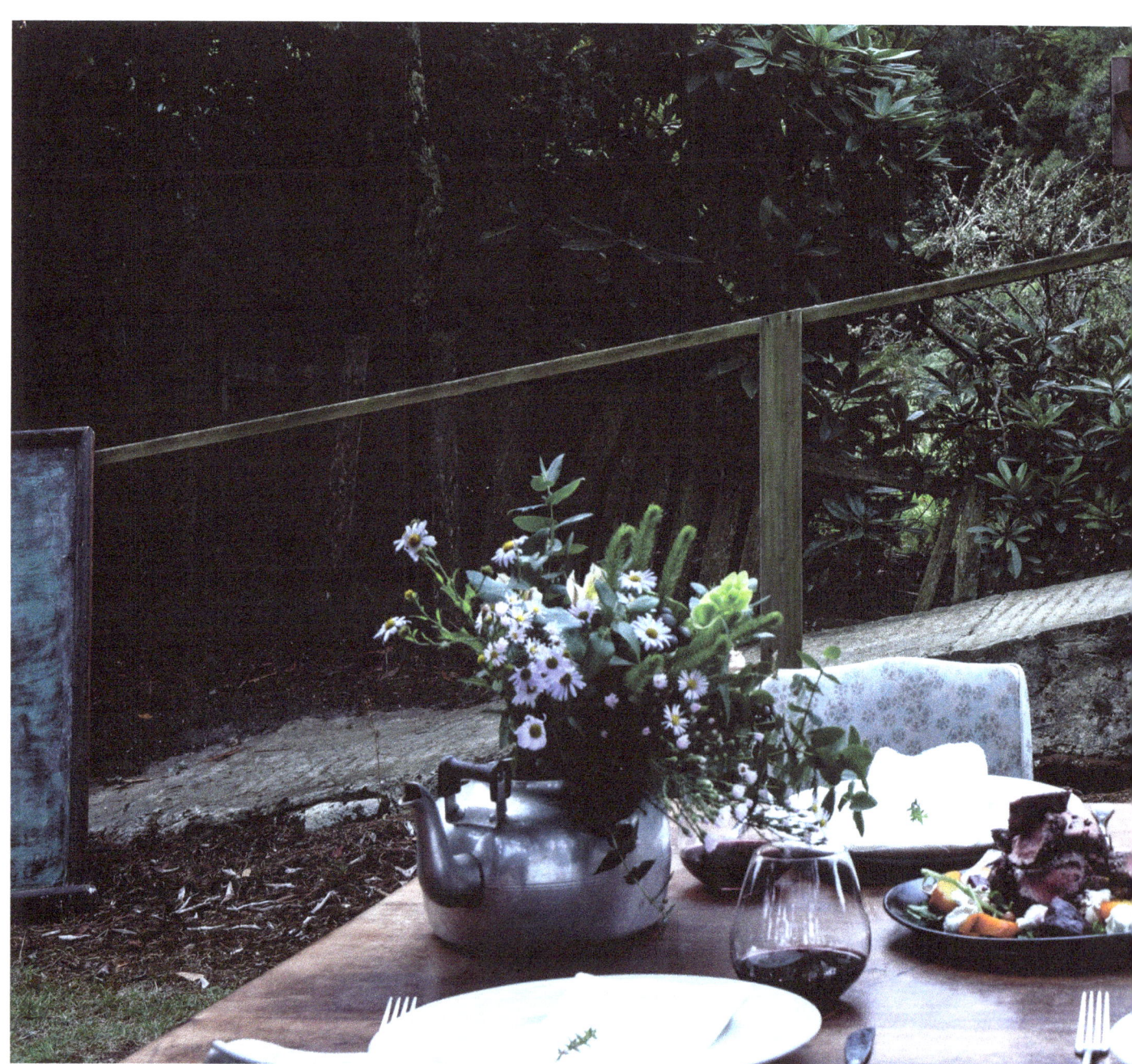

Premium Species

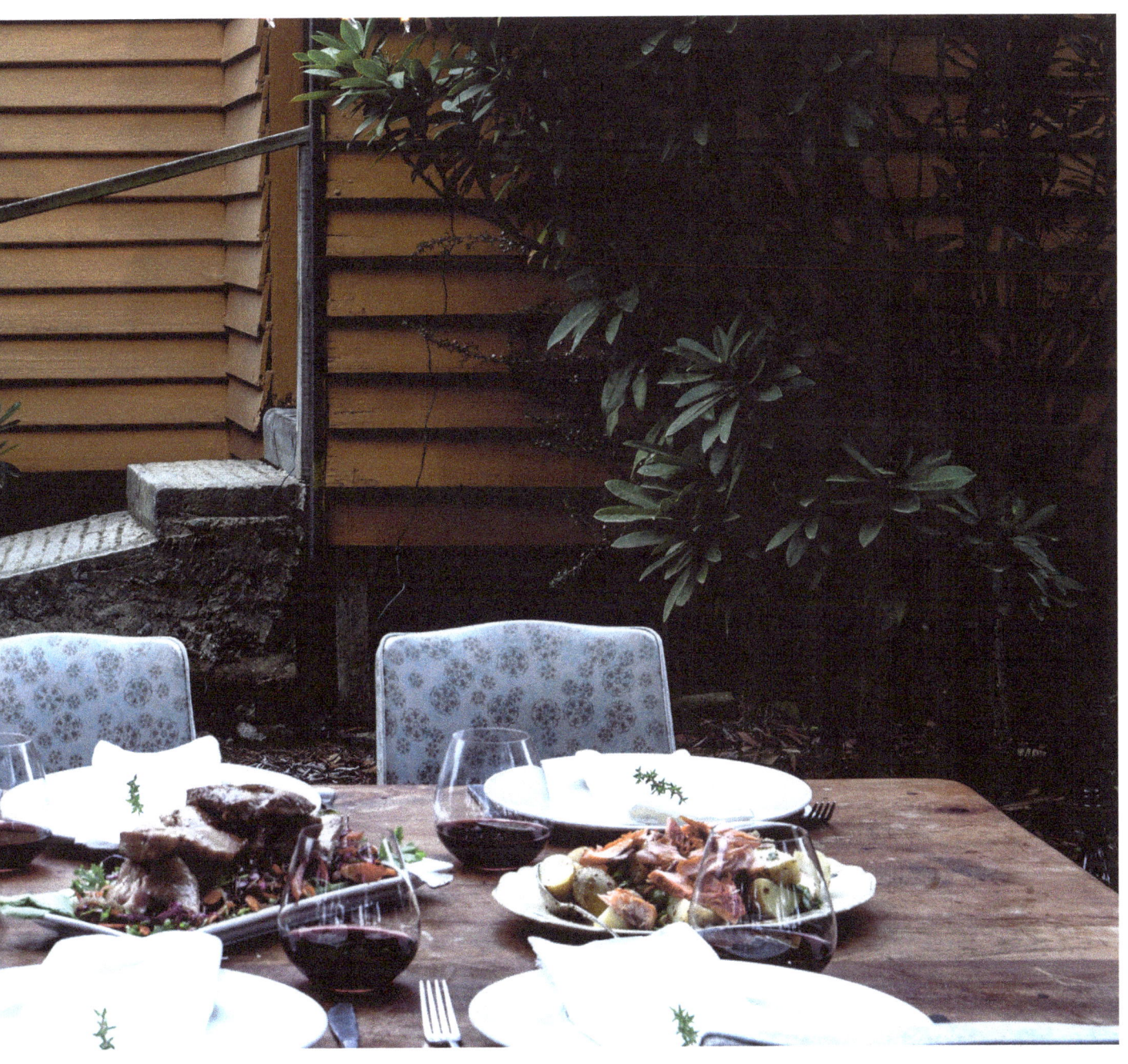

Lemon and Oregano Fish with Fresh Burghul Salad

SERVES 4

Burghul is also known as cracked wheat and is commonly used in Middle Eastern salads such as tabouli. You could also try using cooked rice or cous cous in place of the burghul – the textures would be slightly different but the flavours would still be delicious.

BURGHUL SALAD

1 cup burghul wheat

1 cup peas

½ cup parsley

½ cup mint

1 wedge preserved lemon

2 spring onions

1 cup silver beet or spinach

2 medium carrots

2 cloves garlic

salt and pepper

1 tablespoon extra virgin olive oil

DRESSING

2 tablespoons oregano

1 tablespoon extra virgin olive oil

1 tablespoon lemon juice

FISH

800 grams fish fillets

3 tablespoons flour

salt and pepper

1 teaspoon extra virgin olive oil

1 teaspoon butter

To make the salad, put the burghul into a bowl and cover with boiling water. Set aside for 10 minutes and then drain well by squeezing through a cloth (such as kitchen muslin or a tea towel) to remove all excess water. Bring a small saucepan of water to the boil and cook the peas for one minute, drain and set aside to cool. Finely chop the parsley, mint, preserved lemon, spring onions and silver beet. Grate the carrot and crush the garlic. Add the vegetables to the well-drained burghul, stir through the extra virgin olive oil and season with salt and pepper to taste.

To make the salad dressing, finely chop the oregano and mix with the extra virgin olive oil and lemon juice. Pour half of the dressing over the salad, reserve the remainder for the fish.

To cook the fish, place flour onto a plate and season well with salt and pepper. Press each side of the fish fillets into the flour mixture so they are well coated. Heat a frying pan over moderate heat, add the oil and butter, and cook the fish for about 4 minutes on each side or until golden brown and cooked through.

Pour the dressing over the hot fish and serve immediately with the burghul salad.

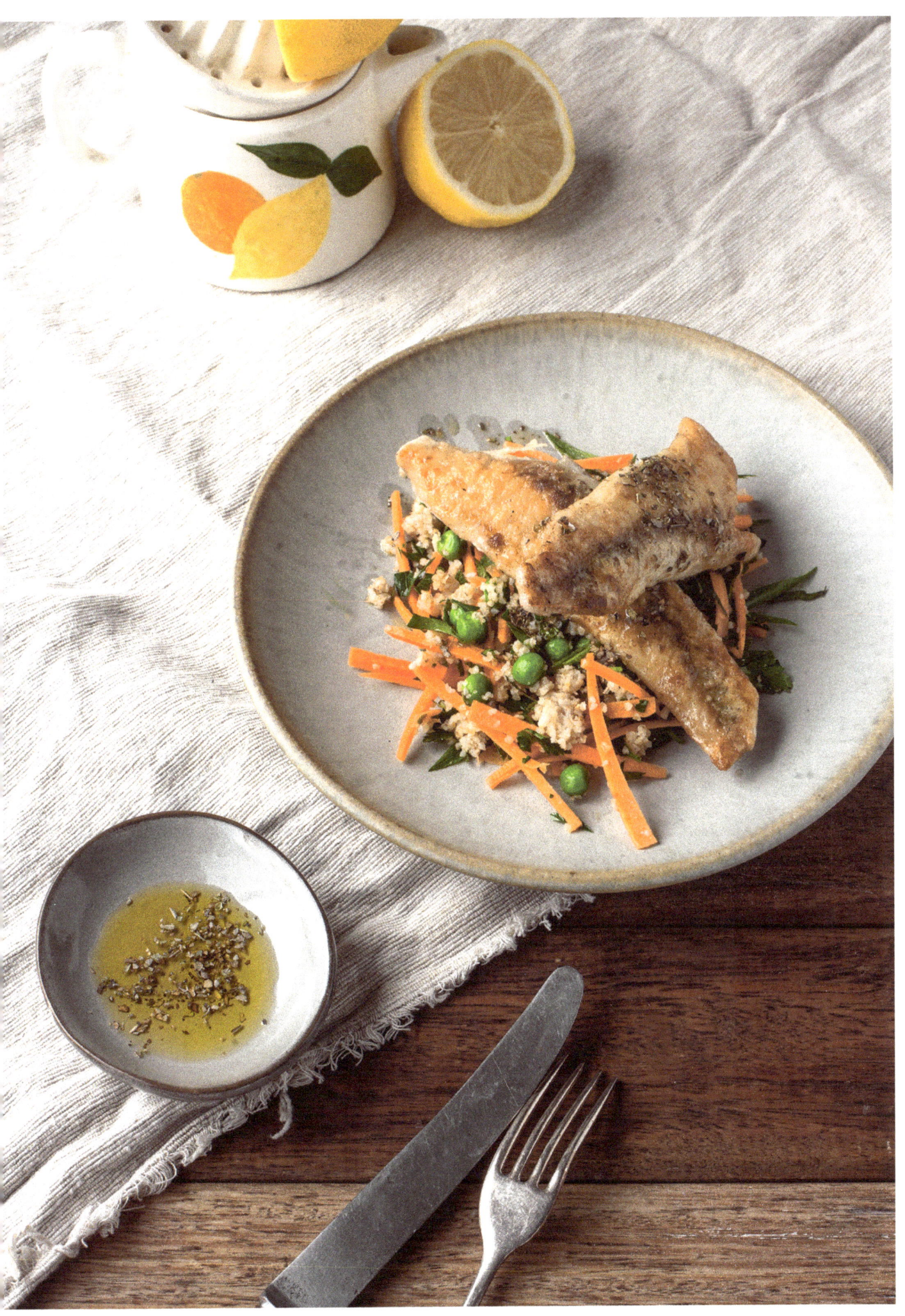

Chilli Salted Fish with Spring Vegetable Risotto

SERVES 4

Bay Trumpeter is a strongly flavoured, white-fleshed fish, and the meat flakes away from the bone when cooked.

RISOTTO

4 ½ cups fish or vegetable stock

1 medium onion

2 cloves garlic

1 tablespoon butter

1 tablespoon extra virgin olive oil

1 cup Arborio rice

1 cup white wine

2 lemons

½ cup parmesan

50 ml cream

1 cup spinach

1 cup peas

½ cup cream

CHILLI SALTED FISH

2 tablespoons sea salt flakes

1 teaspoon chilli flakes

4 x 200 gram pieces fresh fish

1 tablespoon extra virgin olive oil

To make the risotto, bring the stock to the boil in a saucepan, and reduce the heat slightly to keep at a slow boil. Finely dice the onion and garlic. In a large, heavy-based saucepan, melt the butter over medium heat, add the oil and sauté the onion and garlic for a few minutes, until the onion is translucent.

Add the rice and continue to sauté over low heat for 2 minutes. Increase to a medium heat, add the wine and one cup of hot stock, stirring continuously. When the liquid is almost absorbed, add another cup of the stock.

Continue to add the stock in this manner, until it is all used and the rice is very nearly cooked. This will take approximately 25 minutes. Zest and juice the lemon, grate the cheese and stir through the risotto, along with the cream, peas and spinach.

To cook the fish, mix the salt and chilli flakes together in a plastic bag, add the fish and shake to coat. Heat the oil in a frying pan over medium heat, and pan fry the fish for approximately 4 minutes on each side. Serve the fish with the risotto.

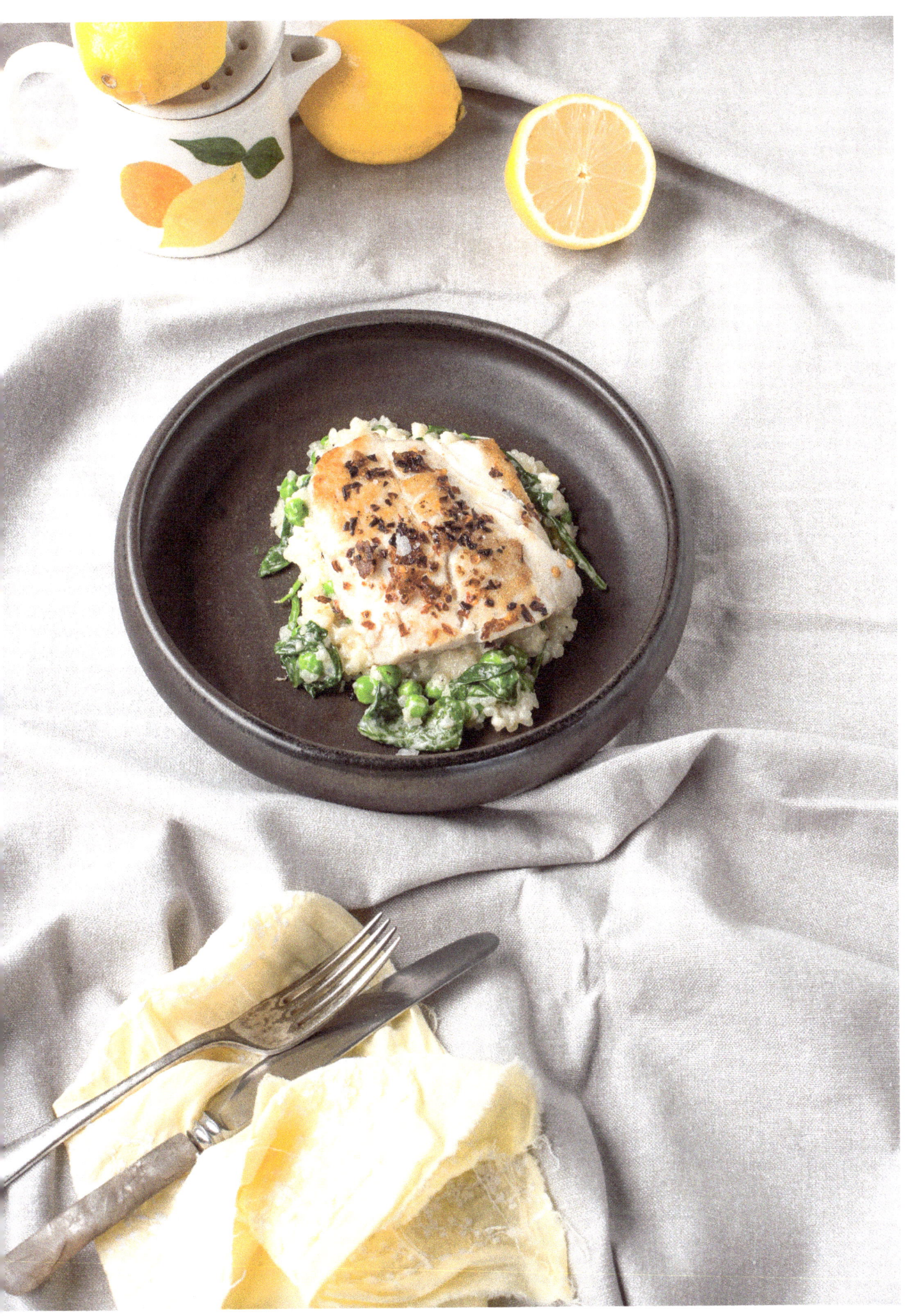

Baked Fish with a Gremolata Crust, Caper Potato Mash and Lemon Butter

SERVES 4

The crust for this dish is a resourceful way to use up crusts and stale bread. Keep a store of these in the freezer until required.

MASHED POTATO

4 large Kennebec potatoes

20 grams butter (150 grams total recipe)

50ml cream (70ml total recipe)

60 grams capers

salt and pepper

GREMOLATA CRUST

4 thick slices of bread

2 wedges of preserved lemon (or zest and 1 tablespoon of juice)

¼ cup mint

¼ cup parsley

1 clove garlic

salt and pepper

40 grams butter

4 x 200 gram pieces of fish

30 grams butter for cooking

LEMON BUTTER SAUCE

juice of one lemon

¼ cup cream

¼ cup white wine

60 grams butter

salt and pepper

Preheat the oven to 180°C. Remove the skin and bones from the fish pieces.

Peel the potatoes and chop into 3cm dice. Place the potatoes in a saucepan of cold water, bring to the boil and cook for 15-20 minutes or until tender. Drain the potatoes well, mash with the butter and cream, stir through the capers and season with salt and pepper.

To make the gremolata crust, roughly chop the bread, blitz in the food processor until crumbs are formed, remove from the processor and set aside. Blend the preserved lemon, mint, parsley, garlic, butter and salt and pepper in the food processor. Return the crumbs to the processor and blitz to combine. Press a ½ cm thick layer of the crumb mix onto each piece of fish. Line an ovenproof tray with baking paper. Cut butter into four portions and place on baking paper. Put each piece of fish, crust side down, on a lump of butter. Bake for approximately 15 minutes until the fish is cooked.

To make the sauce, gently simmer the lemon juice, cream and wine in a small saucepan over low heat until slightly reduced. Remove the pan from heat and whisk in butter until combined. Season to taste with salt and pepper.

To serve, drizzle the sauce over the fish and serve immediately.

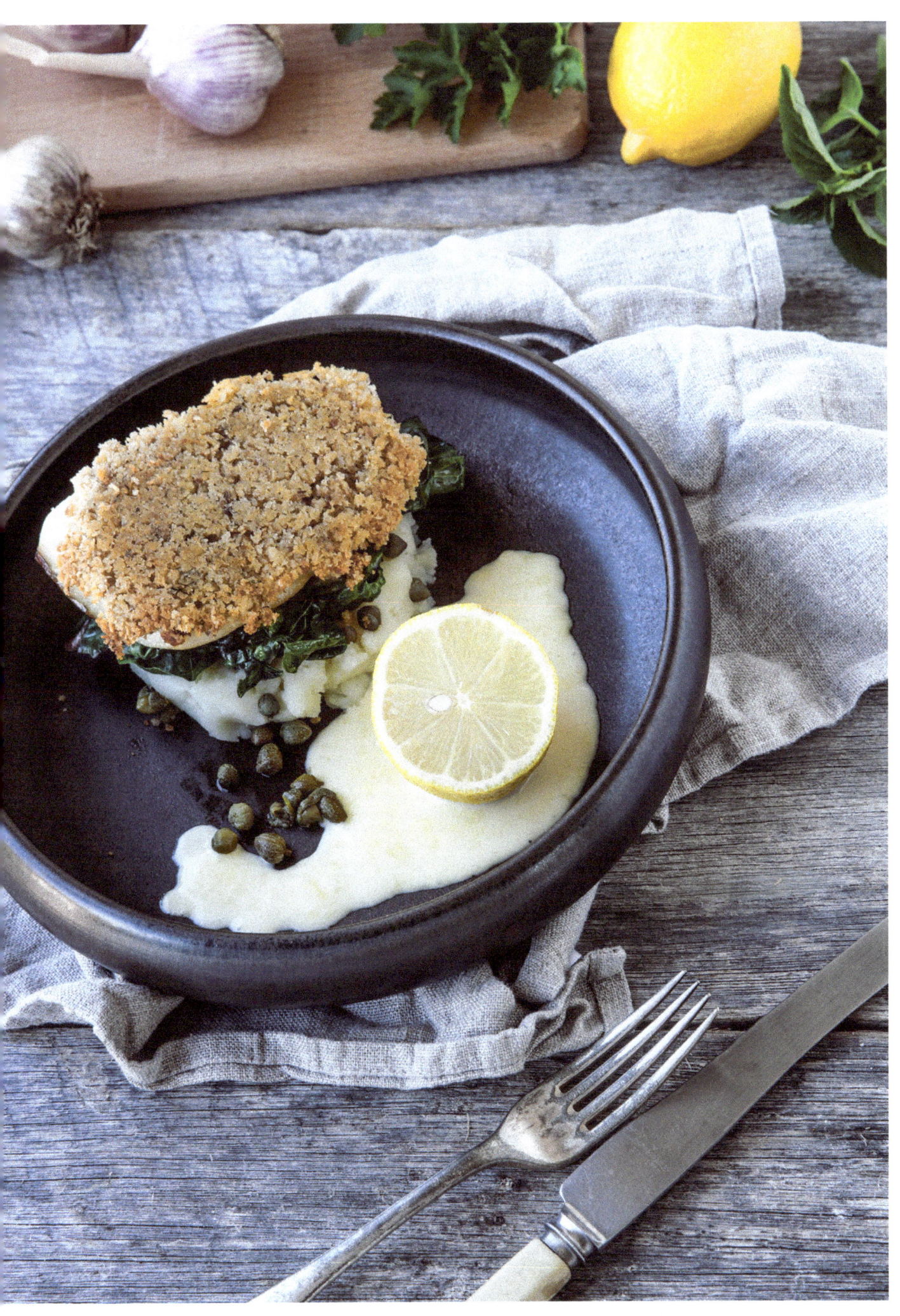

Soy and Balsamic Marinated Fish

SERVES 4

Serve this dish with rice and a crisp green salad.

2 cloves garlic

1 teaspoon fresh ginger

1 tablespoon dill

1 tablespoon soy sauce

1 tablespoon balsamic vinegar

1 tablespoon lime juice

1 tablespoon sesame oil

600 grams skinned and boneless fish fillet

2 tablespoons extra virgin olive oil

To make the marinade, crush the garlic, finely grate the ginger, finely chop the dill and mix well with the soy sauce, balsamic vinegar, lime juice and sesame oil. Slice the fish fillet into steaks 1cm thick. Coat both sides of the fish fillets in the marinade, place in the refrigerator and leave to marinate for at least 2 hours.

To cook the fish, heat the extra virgin olive oil in a frying pan over medium heat, and cook the fish fillets for a few minutes on each side, or until cooked through to your liking. Serve immediately.

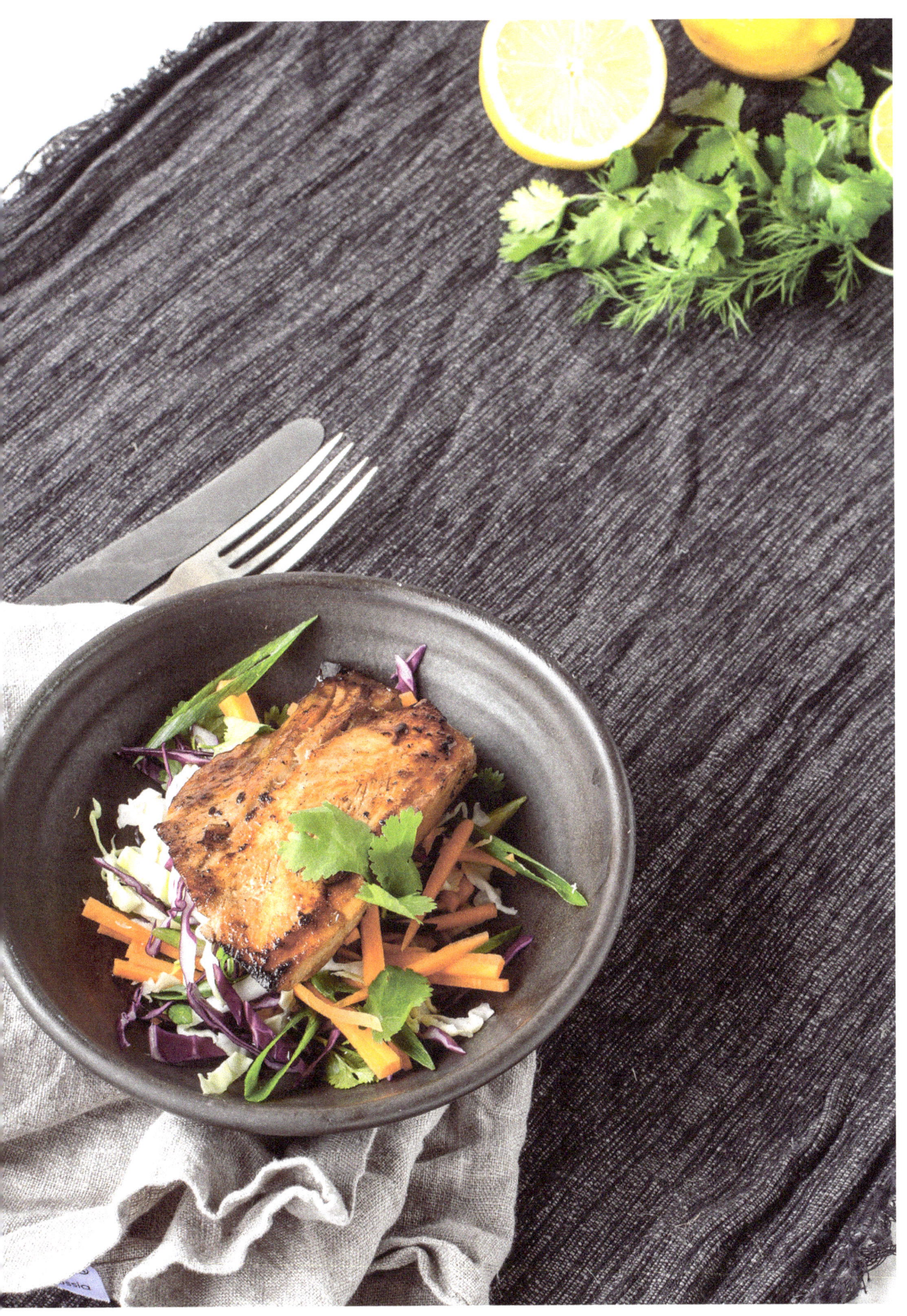

Fish Baked with Tomato, Garlic and Lemon with Homemade Gnocchi

SERVES 4

If you haven't tried making gnocchi before, this method is fast, easy and works a treat, resulting in soft, fluffy gnocchi. Combined with brown butter, garlic and sage it's delicious combination and one you will find yourself returning to again and again. The gnocchi can be made in advance and reheated quickly in boiling water when required.

GNOCCHI

500 grams Kennebec potatoes

2 eggs

salt and pepper

1 cup flour

pinch nutmeg

BAKED FISH

800 grams fish

2 tomatoes

1 lemon

1 Spanish onion

2 teaspoons garlic

salt and pepper

2 teaspoons extra virgin olive oil

4 tablespoons fresh basil

GNOCCHI SAUCE

3 tablespoons butter

2 tablespoons garlic

2 tablespoons fresh sage

2 cups baby spinach leaves

salt and pepper

1 cup shaved parmesan

To make the gnocchi, peel and dice the potatoes into 2cm cubes. Place potatoes in a saucepan, cover with water, bring to the boil and simmer for 18 minutes or until the potatoes are cooked through. Drain well and set aside to cool for a few minutes. While the potatoes are still warm, mash well and stir through the eggs, nutmeg, flour and a pinch of salt and pepper. If the dough is too sticky to handle, add a little more flour. Using lightly floured hands, roll the dough into balls around the size of a ten cent piece, and set aside on a lightly floured plate until ready to cook.

To cook the gnocchi, bring a large pot of salted water to the boil. Carefully place the gnocchi into the water and bring back to a simmer. Continue to simmer for about 4 minutes, or until cooked through, drain and set aside until ready to use.

To cook the fish, pre-heat the oven to 180°C. Cut out four pieces of tinfoil, and four pieces of greaseproof paper, into squares 20cm x 20cm in size. Lay the pieces of greaseproof paper on top of the foil. Cut the fish into 4 equal portions and lay a piece of fish on top of each piece of paper/foil. Slice the tomato, lemon and onion, crush the garlic and combine with the salt, pepper, oil and chopped basil, and top each piece of fish with this mixture. Fold up the edges of the parcel tightly to fully enclose the fish. Place the parcels on a baking tray and cook for about 15 minutes or until the fish is cooked to your liking.

To serve, heat a large frying pan over high heat and add the butter. When the butter starts to froth, add the crushed garlic. When the garlic browns, reduce the heat to medium and add the finely chopped sage, spinach leaves and gnocchi. Season to taste and gently stir to coat all of the gnocchi in the butter mixture. Serve the gnocchi with the baked fish and top with shaved parmesan cheese.

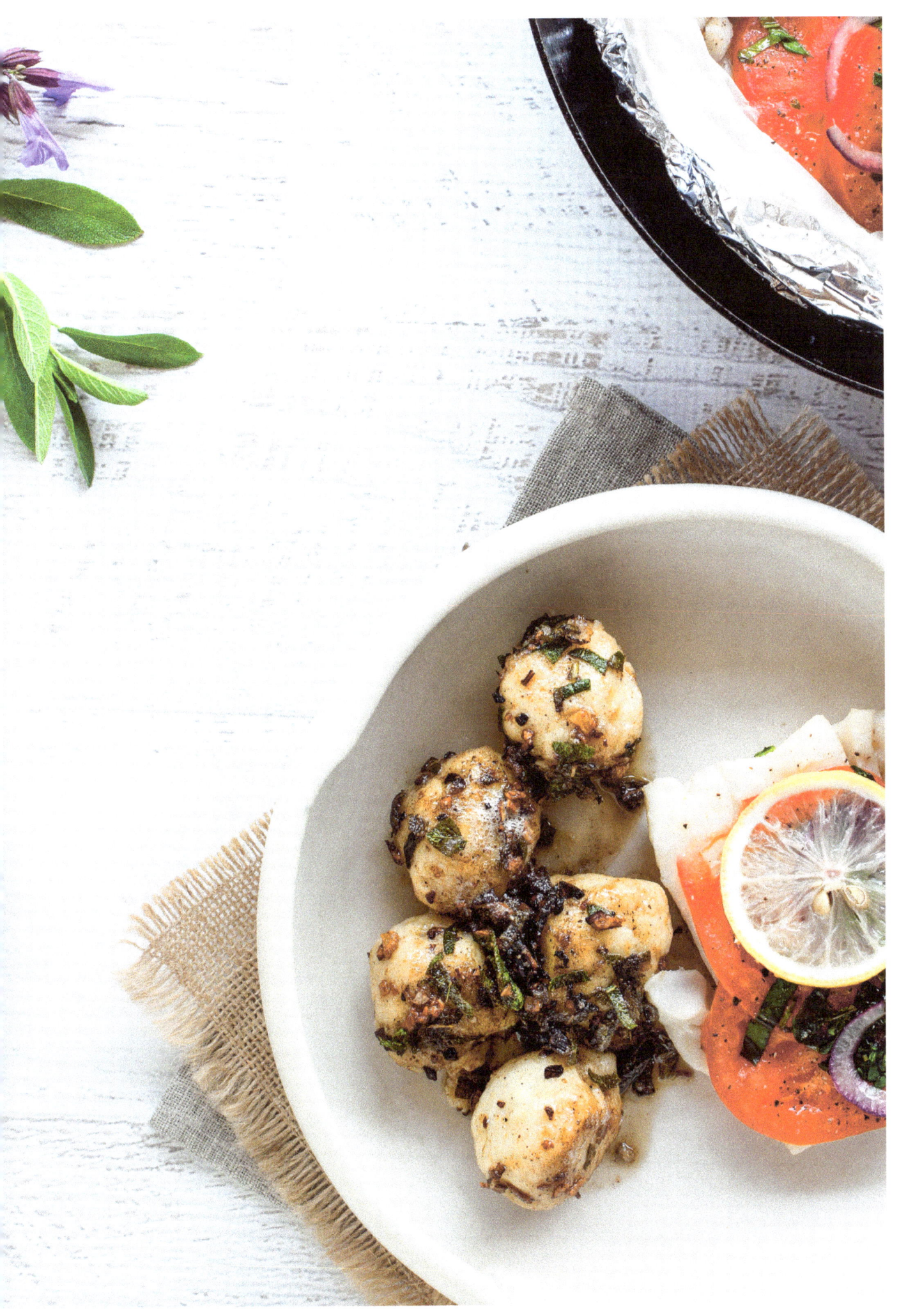

Peppered Tuna Steak with a Warm Marinated Vegetable Salad and Grilled Kefalograviera Cheese

SERVES 4

The recipe for this salad is very adaptable - I like to make it with what I have available at home and I often add cooked or marinated mushrooms, fresh or dried tomatoes or other seasonal vegetables. Kefalograviera is a Greek cheese which is suitable for grilling or frying, and halloumi cheese could be substituted if necessary. If you are not topping the tuna with the Kefalograviera, you could toss goat's cheese or feta through the salad instead.

SALAD

1 large eggplant

½ teaspoon sea salt

2 medium zucchini

extra virgin olive oil

2 large red capsicums

1 cup spinach leaves

2 tablespoons shredded basil

100 grams black pitted olives

TUNA

4 tuna steaks, 600-800 grams total

1 tablespoon black peppercorns

1 tablespoon native pepper berries

1 tablespoon fennel seed

2 tablespoons salt

CHEESE

200 grams Kefalograviera cheese (or halloumi cheese)

60ml extra virgin olive oil

2 tablespoons plain flour

TO SERVE

2 lemons

Pre-heat the oven to 200°C.

To prepare the salad, slice eggplant into 1cm rounds, sprinkle both sides with salt and set aside for one hour. This will remove any bitter flavours from the eggplant. Rinse well under cold water and drain well. Slice the zucchini lengthways into 1cm strips. Brush the zucchini and eggplant with extra virgin olive oil and pan fry, barbeque or grill using medium heat, until cooked through. Dice into 1cm pieces. Brush the red capsicum with oil and roast in the hot oven for 20 minutes. Remove from the oven and place in a bowl. Cover with plastic wrap and set aside to cool. When cool enough to handle, peel off and discard the skin and seeds. Chop the capsicum flesh into 1cm dice.

When ready to serve the salad, heat a dash of extra virgin olive oil in a frying pan over low heat, and toss the zucchini, eggplant and capsicum together. Stir through the spinach, basil and olives.

To prepare the tuna, remove the tuna steaks from the refrigerator to come to room temperature. Make the pepper coating for the tuna by sprinkling the black peppercorns, pepper berries and fennel seed onto a baking tray, and roasting for 10 minutes. Remove from the oven and cool. Using a food processor, or mortar and pestle, grind the roasted spices and salt to a fine powder. Roll each tuna steak in the pepper mix to coat.

To cook the tuna, pre-heat the grill, barbeque or frying pan over medium-high heat. Cook the tuna steaks for 2-3 minutes on each side, or until cooked to your liking (for thicker steaks this timing will result in rare tuna steaks).

To cook the Kefalograviera, slice the cheese into ½ cm pieces. Coat the cheese in flour, and heat the extra virgin olive oil in a frying pan (or the flat plate of a barbeque) over medium-high heat. Cook the cheese pieces for 1-2 minutes on each side, or until golden and crisp on the outside, and soft and gooey in the middle.

To serve, place a tuna steak on top of the warmed salad and top with the cheese. Slice the lemons in half and serve each plate with half a lemon to squeeze over the top.

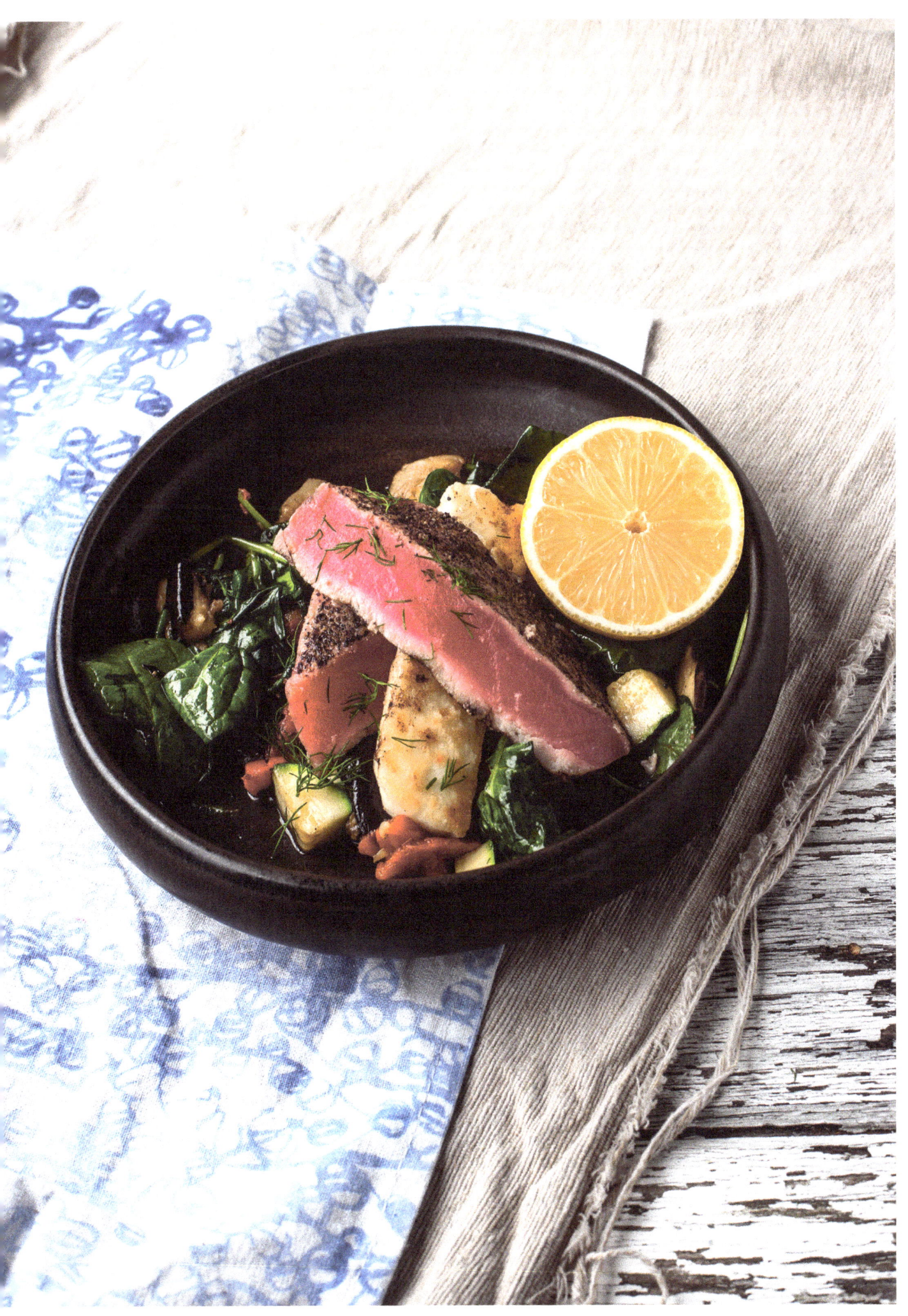

Pan-fried Fish with a Blue Cheese and Potato Gratin and Cauliflower Puree

SERVES 4

POTATO GRATIN

600 grams Kennebec potatoes

1 medium sweet potato

1 small onion

200 grams blue cheese

½ cup parmesan cheese

1 egg

1 cup stock

1 cup cream

60 grams butter

salt and pepper

CAULIFLOWER PUREE

2 cups cauliflower florets

½ cup cream

1 clove garlic

salt and pepper

PAN-FRIED FLATHEAD

800 grams fish fillets

2 tablespoons plain flour

salt and pepper

2 tablespoons extra virgin olive oil

1 tablespoon butter

Pre-heat the oven to 180°C.

To make the gratin, peel the potatoes, sweet potato and onion and finely slice into 2mm rounds. Crumble the blue cheese and grate the parmesan cheese. Using a small baking tray, create layers of potato, onion and then blue cheese. Use the sweet potato to create the middle layer, and top with more layers of the potato, onion and blue cheese. Whisk together the egg, stock, cream and parmesan cheese in a small bowl and pour the mixture over the gratin. Slice the butter and distribute evenly over the top of the gratin as the final layer. Cover with foil and bake for 1 hour, or until cooked through when tested with a sharp knife. Remove from the oven to rest, and compress the gratin by placing a smaller baking tray or board on top of the cooked gratin, and placing a stack of plates or some tins on top for additional weight.

To make the cauliflower puree, bring a large saucepan of water to the boil, and cut the cauliflower into 2cm pieces. Cook the cauliflower in the boiling water for 10 minutes or until tender. Drain the cauliflower and use a food processor (or stick blender) to puree with the cream and garlic, adding salt and pepper to taste.

To cook the fish, remove the skin and bones from the fish fillets. Season the flour with salt and pepper, sprinkle onto a plate and roll the fish in the flour. Heat the oil and butter in a frying pan over medium heat, and pan fry the fish for a few minutes on each side, until cooked to your liking.

Serve the fish fillets with the gratin and cauliflower puree.

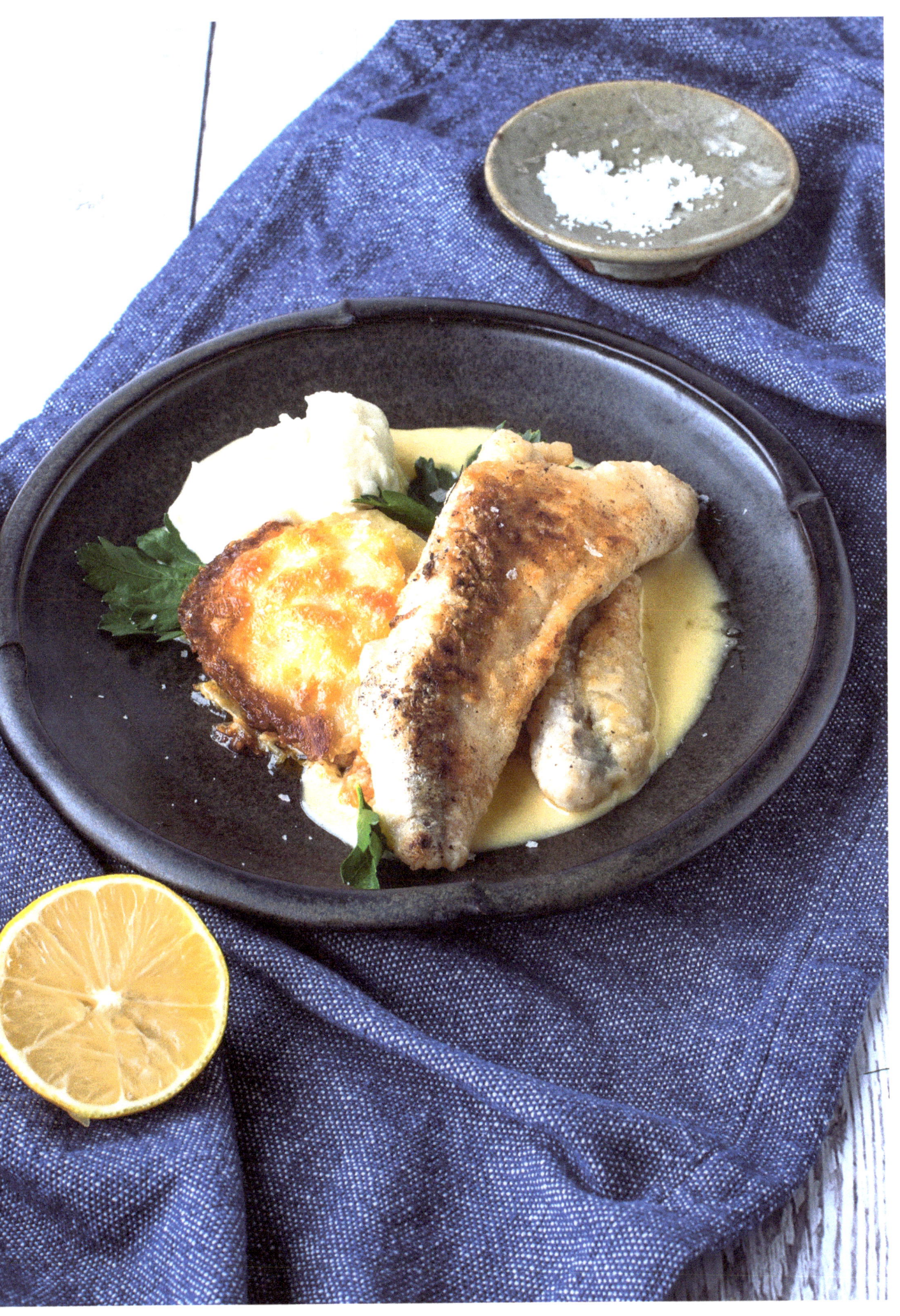

Macadamia Crusted Fish with Wasabi Potato Mash and Beetroot and Lime Chutney

SERVES 4

This delicious dish is wonderful to share with friends and is ideally served with sautéed seasonal greens. Wasabi paste is available from supermarkets and can be very hot, so add it gradually and taste as you go to ensure the mash is to your liking!

WASABI MASH

4 large Kennebec potatoes

30 grams butter

30ml cream

10 grams wasabi paste (or to your liking)

salt and pepper

CRUSTED FISH

4 slices white bread

50 grams macadamia nuts

15 grams fresh ginger

1 clove garlic

50 grams butter

salt and pepper

4 pieces of fish (180-200 grams each)

40 grams butter

BEETROOT AND LIME CHUTNEY

2 medium beetroot

½ Spanish onion

1 lemon

3 limes

1 tablespoon sugar

15ml vinegar

Pre-heat the oven to 180°C.

To make the mash, peel and dice the potatoes. Put potatoes into a large saucepan, cover with water, bring to the boil and cook for 15-20 minutes or until cooked through. Drain well and mash with the butter and cream. Stir through the wasabi and season to taste with salt and pepper.

To make the macadamia crust, roughly chop the bread and use a food processor to process into breadcrumbs. Remove from the processor and set aside. Add the macadamias, grated ginger, garlic, butter, salt and pepper and process until well combined. Add the breadcrumbs to the processor, pulse to combine. Spread a ½ cm thick layer of the mixture on top of each piece of fish.

To cook the fish, slice the butter into 4 pieces. Line a baking dish with baking paper. Place the crusted fish pieces on top of a piece of butter, crust side down. Bake for 15 minutes, or until the fish is cooked through.

To make the chutney, peel and grate the beetroot, finely slice the onion, zest and the juice the lemons and limes. Using a small saucepan, combine the sugar, vinegar, beetroot, onion, zest and juice and simmer over medium heat for 15 minutes, or until the beetroot is cooked and soft. Remove from heat and set aside.

To serve, top the mash with a piece of fish and a dollop of beetroot chutney.

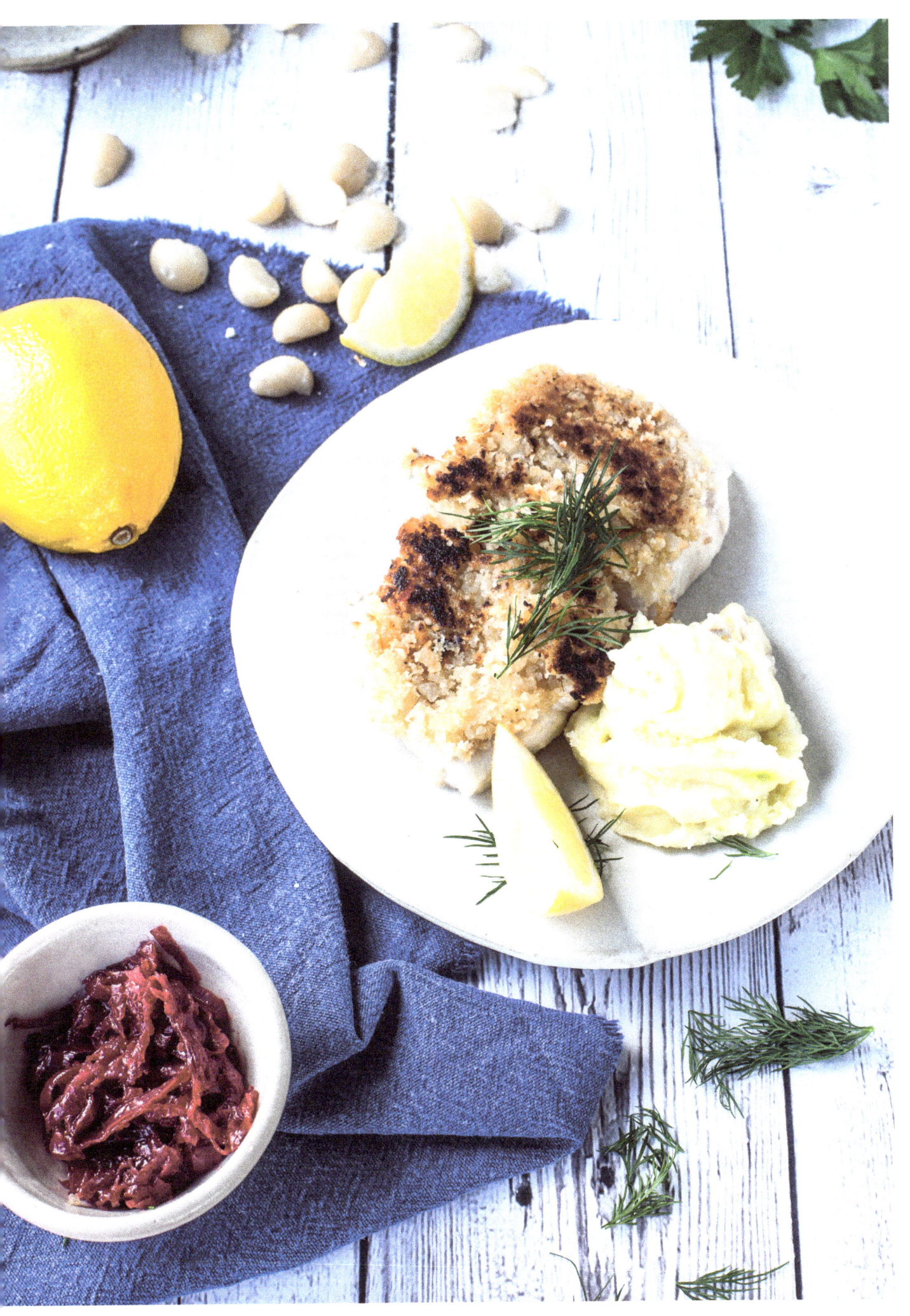

Salmon Poached in a Thyme and Mushroom Cream Sauce

SERVES 4

If you don't have the time to make your own pasta for this dish, dried pasta works perfectly well. Simply cook to the packet instructions and continue with the dish.

FETTUCCINI

200 grams plain flour

1 tablespoon extra virgin olive oil

2 eggs

SALMON IN CREAM SAUCE

1 brown onion

3 cloves garlic

1 cup mushrooms

1 tablespoon basil

1 tablespoon extra virgin olive oil

½ cup white wine

2 cups cream

4 salmon steaks, (180-200 grams each, skinless and boneless)

5 sprigs fresh thyme

salt and pepper

1 cup parmesan cheese

Use a food processor to make the pasta dough. Place the flour in the food processor. Turn on the processor and with the motor running, add the extra virgin olive oil and the eggs. Continue blending until the mixture comes together to form a firm dough. If the mixture seems too wet or sticky to handle, knead in a little more flour by hand on a floured bench.

To roll the pasta, divide the dough into 4 portions. Using a pasta machine set at number 1 (or at the widest setting) feed each portion of the dough through the machine. Repeat this process with each portion of pasta on each setting, until you reach setting number 6, (or the highest setting on your machine) the pasta should be 2mm thick, silky smooth and slightly elastic.

Cut the pasta into fettuccini strips using the appropriate cutter on the pasta machine. Dust the bench with flour and carefully lay the lengths of dough aside until needed.

To make the salmon in cream sauce, dice the onion, crush the garlic and slice the mushrooms. Chop the basil. Heat the extra virgin olive oil over medium heat in a large, heavy-based frying pan, and sauté the onion, garlic and mushrooms for 2 minutes or until softened and well cooked.

Deglaze the pan with the wine and then add the cream and salmon steaks. Turn the heat to low and simmer to reduce the sauce. If the sauce starts to reduce too much while the salmon is cooking, add a little more wine or cream. Alternatively, if the salmon is cooked before the sauce has reduced, remove the salmon from the pan and return once the sauce is to your liking.

To finish, add the thyme and basil, and season with salt and pepper to taste. When the salmon is almost cooked, add the pre-cooked fettuccini to the sauce to heat through. Serve the fettuccini and cream sauce topped with a salmon steak and sprinkled with shaved parmesan cheese.

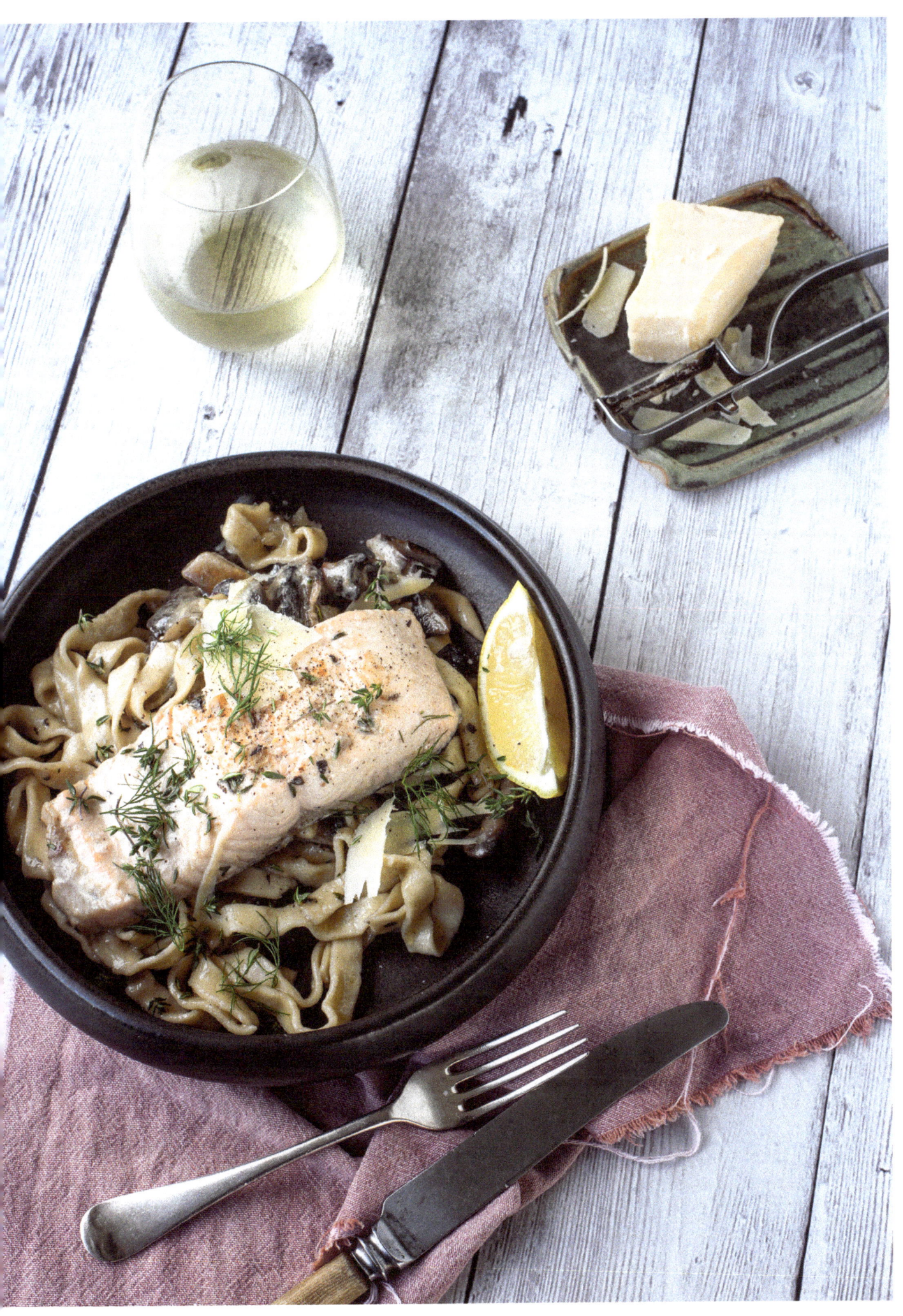

Five Spice Poached Coconut Salmon

SERVES 4

Roasting your own spices for the five spice mix intensifies the flavours, and gives this dish a wonderful depth.

FIVE SPICE MIX

1 teaspoon Sichuan pepper

1 teaspoon star anise

1 teaspoon fennel seed

1 cinnamon stick
(or 1 teaspoon ground cinnamon)

1 teaspoon cloves

1 packet rice noodles (or 4 servings)

POACHED SALMON

1 tablespoon extra virgin olive oil

1 medium onion

500ml vegetable or fish stock

1 litre coconut milk

20ml fish sauce

1 tablespoon palm sugar

1 tablespoon lime juice

4 x 180-200 gram salmon steaks
(skinless and boneless)

1 bunch bok choy

2 tablespoons coriander

salt and pepper

Pre-heat the oven to 180°C.

To make the five spice powder, sprinkle the spices onto a baking tray and roast in the oven for 10 minutes. Remove from the oven, cool and grind to a fine powder using a mortar and pestle or food processor.

Cook the rice noodles, following directions on the packet.

Heat the extra virgin olive oil in a large, heavy-based frying pan over medium heat and sauté the onion for 5 minutes or until softened. Add the five-spice powder, stock, fish sauce, grated palm sugar and lime juice and then the coconut milk.

Bring to a gentle simmer and add the salmon steaks. Poach the salmon until cooked to your liking; 8 minutes will result in medium-rare salmon. Add the cooked rice noodles, chopped coriander leaves and bok choy, and simmer until the noodles have heated through and the bok choy has softened.

Season with salt and pepper to taste and serve immediately.

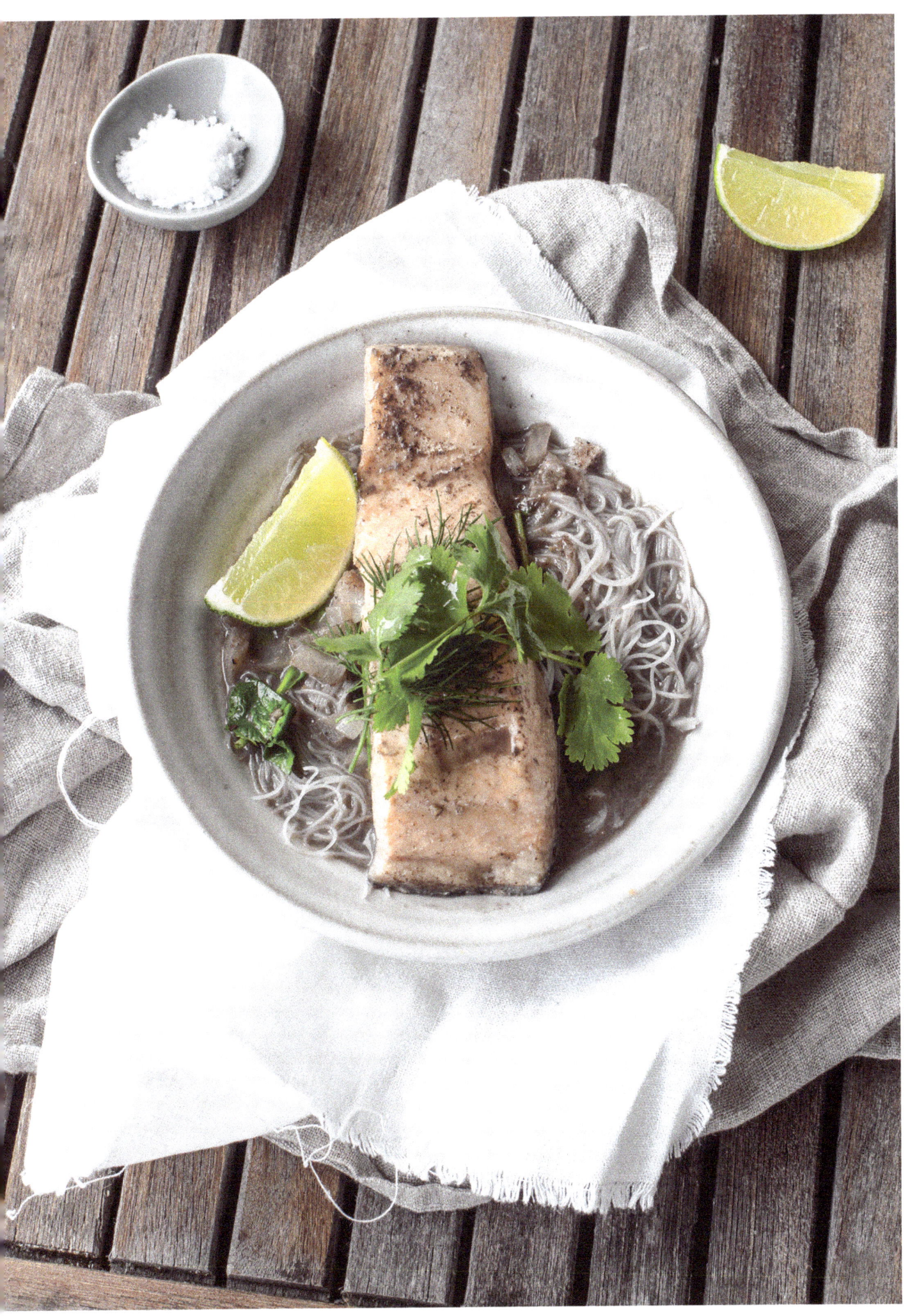

Baked Salmon with Pumpkin Pancakes, Crispy Bacon and Honey Mustard Aioli

SERVES 4

PANCAKES

200 grams pumpkin

1 cup self-raising flour

¾ cup milk

1 egg

1 tablespoon basil

1 clove garlic

salt and pepper

2 tablespoons extra virgin olive oil

1 tablespoon butter

AIOLI

2 egg yolks

1 egg

30ml white vinegar

2 tablespoons honey

1 tablespoon seeded mustard

1 clove garlic

salt and pepper

200ml extra virgin olive oil

BAKED SALMON

4 x 200g salmon steaks (skinless and boneless)

4 large rashers bacon

Pre-heat the oven to 180°C.

To make the pancakes, peel the pumpkin and chop into 1cm dice. Toss the pumpkin in one tablespoon of the extra virgin olive oil, tip onto a baking tray and roast for 30 minutes or until cooked through and golden. Set aside to cool. Whisk together the flour, milk and egg in a large mixing bowl, stir in the shredded basil and crushed garlic and season with salt and pepper. Stir in the roasted pumpkin. Heat the remaining extra virgin olive oil and the butter in a large frying pan over medium heat and drop in tablespoons of batter. Cook the pancakes for 1-2 minutes on each side or until cooked through and golden brown on both sides.

Use a food processor to make the aioli. Blend together the egg yolks, whole egg, vinegar, honey, mustard, crushed garlic and a sprinkle of salt and pepper. With the motor still running, pour the extra virgin olive oil into the processor in a slow drizzle until the aioli is thick and creamy.

To cook the salmon, heat an oven-proof frying pan on the stove top over medium/high heat and quickly seal the flesh side of the salmon pieces. Turn over so the skin side is facing down, add the rashers of bacon to the pan, and put into the oven. Bake until the salmon is cooked to your liking. Cooking for 15 minutes will result in medium salmon.

Serve the salmon with the pumpkin pancakes and a rasher of bacon, with a dollop of honey-mustard aioli.

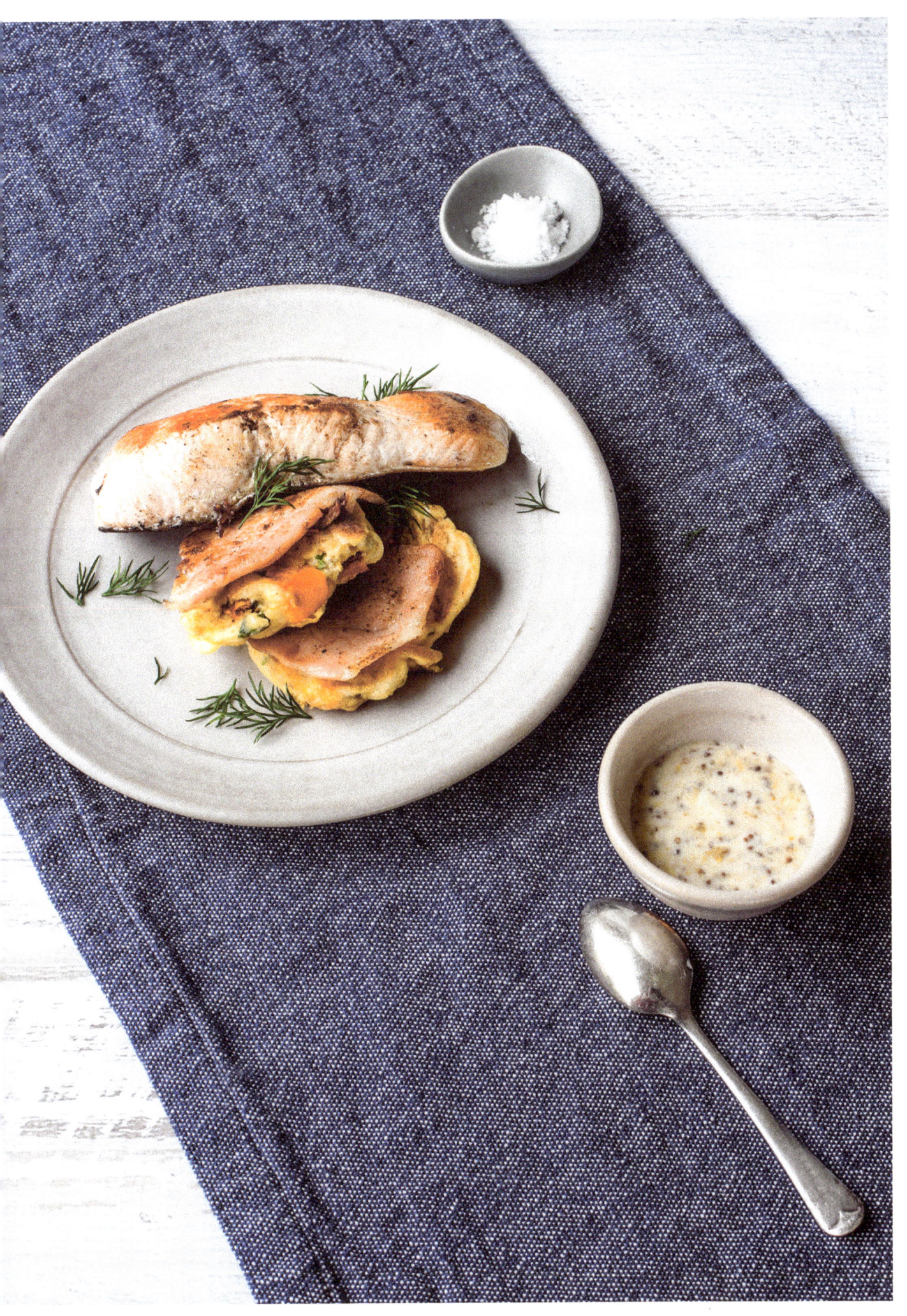

Fish with a Zucchini Salad

SERVES 4

This is a seemingly simple dish, but when you are harvesting in-season tomatoes, zucchini and herbs from your garden, paired with fresh caught fish, dinner doesn't get much better than this!

SALAD

2 large zucchini

1 tablespoon extra virgin olive oil

4 large tomatoes

100 grams feta cheese

1 large clove garlic

1 tablespoon fresh mint

2 tablespoons fresh dill

1 teaspoon lemon juice

1 cup snow peas

salt and pepper

FISH

4 x 200 gram pieces fish

2 tablespoons flour

1 teaspoon extra virgin olive oil

Pre-heat the barbeque grill plate, or a frying pan on the stove top, over medium heat.

To make the salad, slice the zucchini lengthways in 3 mm wide strips. Roll the zucchini slices in a little of the extra virgin olive oil, and grill or pan fry for minute on each side or until cooked through and golden brown. Chop the tomato and feta into 1cm dice, crush the garlic, slice the mint and the dill. Toss together with the remaining extra virgin olive oil, lemon juice, snow peas and the warm zucchini and season with a little salt and pepper.

To cook the fish, season the flour with a little salt and pepper and coat each piece of fish in the flour. Heat the extra virgin olive oil in a heavy-based pan over medium heat. Fry the fish, first skin side up for 2 minutes and finish cooking skin side down for 4 minutes, to create a crispy skin.

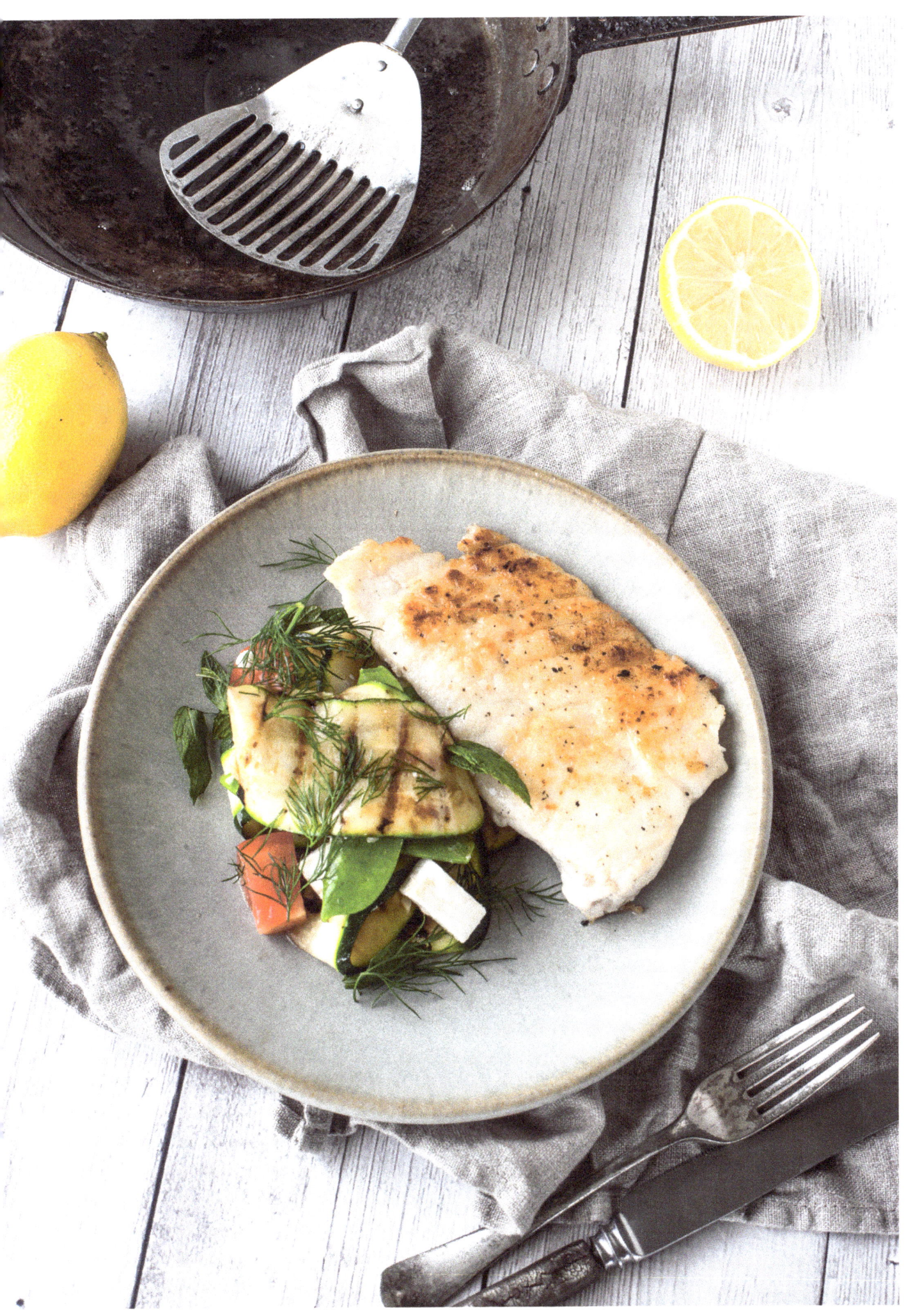

Fish with Peas and Burnt Butter

SERVES 4

If in season, freshly podded peas are a treat and a labour of love! However, frozen peas are a good alternative if fresh peas are unavailable.

2 tablespoons flour

salt and pepper

4 x 150 gram fish fillets

1 tablespoon extra virgin olive oil

2 cups peas

2 tablespoons butter

1 clove garlic

20 sage leaves

To cook the fish, season the flour with a little salt and pepper and coat each piece of fish in the flour. Heat the extra virgin olive oil in a heavy-based frying pan over medium heat.

Cook the fish for one minute on each side, reduce the heat and cook for approximately 4 more minutes (this cooking time is appropriate for fillets of 2cm thickness, adjust the cooking time if necessary).

To cook the peas, bring a saucepan of water to the boil. Dunk the peas in the boiling water for one minute and then drain.

When the fish is cooked, remove the fillets from the pan and set aside to keep warm. Adjust the heat to high, add the butter and crushed garlic to the frying pan and stir until the butter starts to froth and turn brown. Add the chopped sage and peas and stir to coat in the butter mixture.

Serve each piece of fish with the peas and burnt butter.

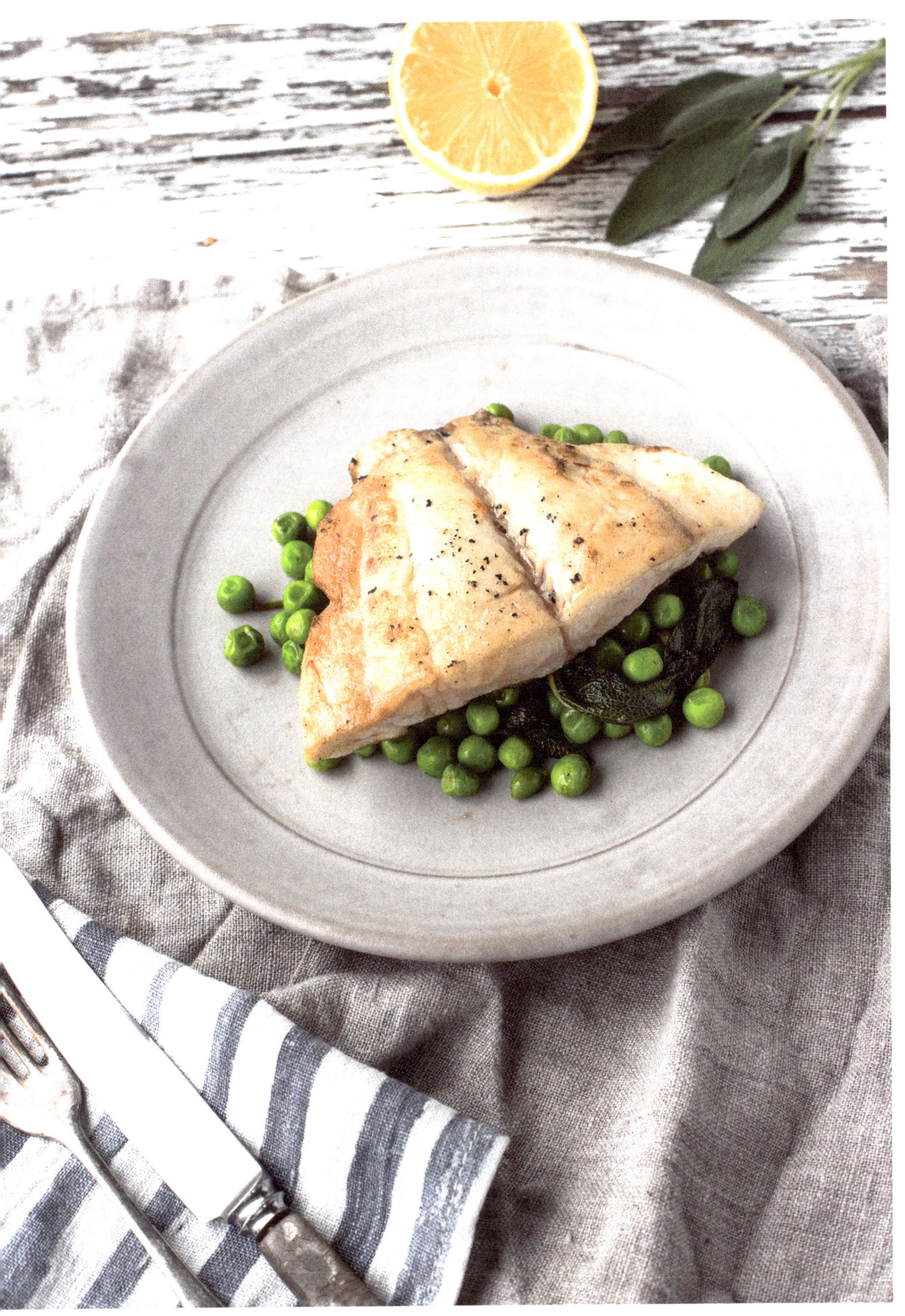

Tuna Carpaccio

SERVES 4 AS AN ENTRÉE, OR LIGHT LUNCH.

Carpaccio is a classic Italian dish. It is best when the tuna is extremely fresh, and even better when caught the same day! Carpaccio is also very simple to make, just take care to use a very sharp knife and slice the tuna as thinly as possible. Although I prefer my tuna carpaccio raw, the fish can be left to marinate in the acidic lemon juice and vinegar to cure slightly if you prefer. You can also try using different vinegars and herbs to create alternate flavours.

320 grams tuna

1 tablespoon red or white wine vinegar

1 tablespoon lemon juice

1 tablespoon capers

1 tablespoon fresh basil, dill and/or parsley

2 tablespoon extra virgin olive oil

sea salt and cracked black pepper

Slice the tuna into very thin slices (each slice should be almost transparent) and arrange on a large platter, or on 4 individual plates. Drizzle the vinegar and lemon juice over the tuna. If you prefer to cure the fish, set it aside for between 10 minutes and one hour until cured to your liking. Finely chop the capers and herbs. Drizzle the tuna with extra virgin olive oil, and sprinkle with the capers, herbs, salt and pepper.

Serve with grissini or crusty bread to mop up the vinegar and extra virgin olive oil.

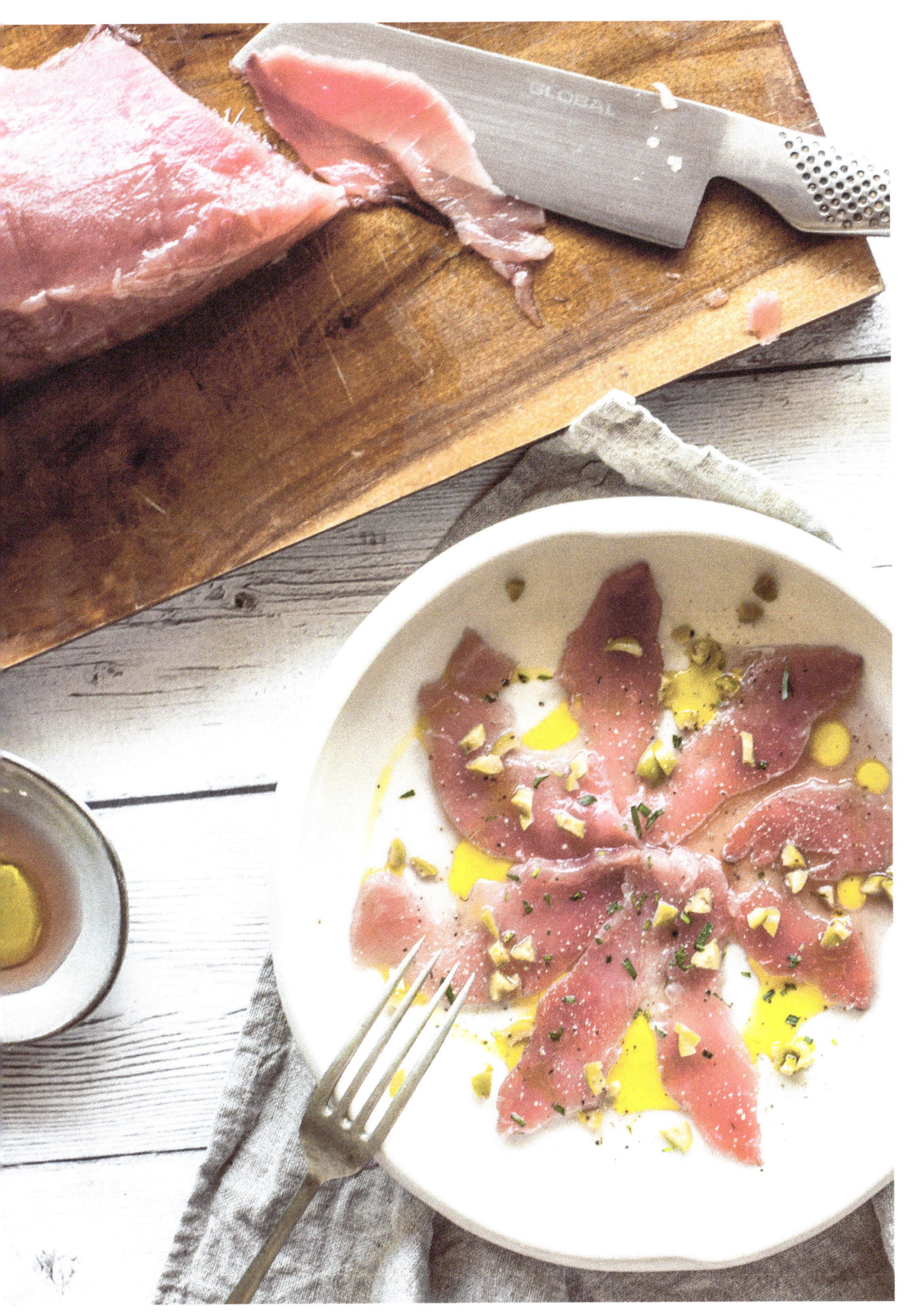

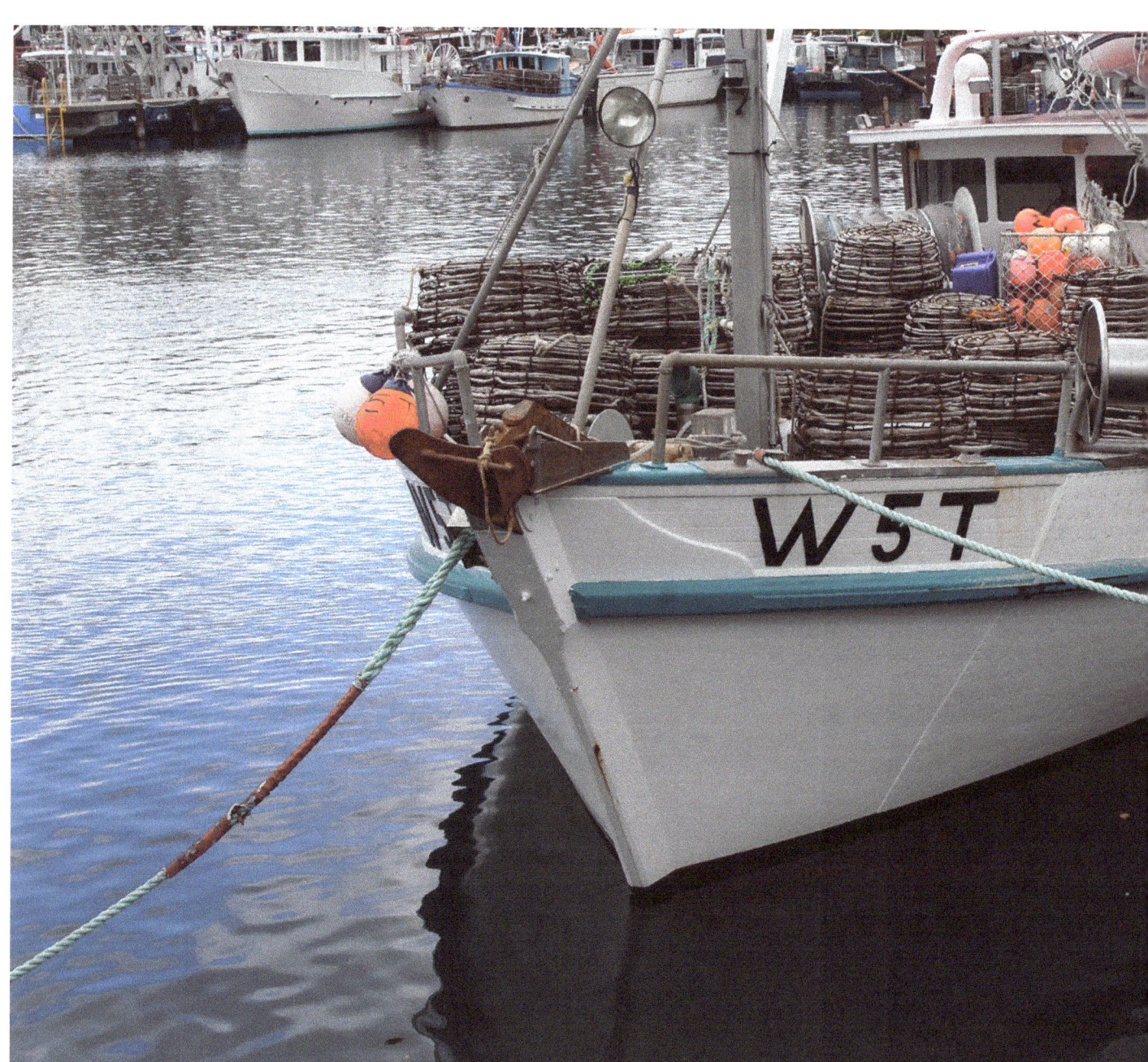

Crayfish

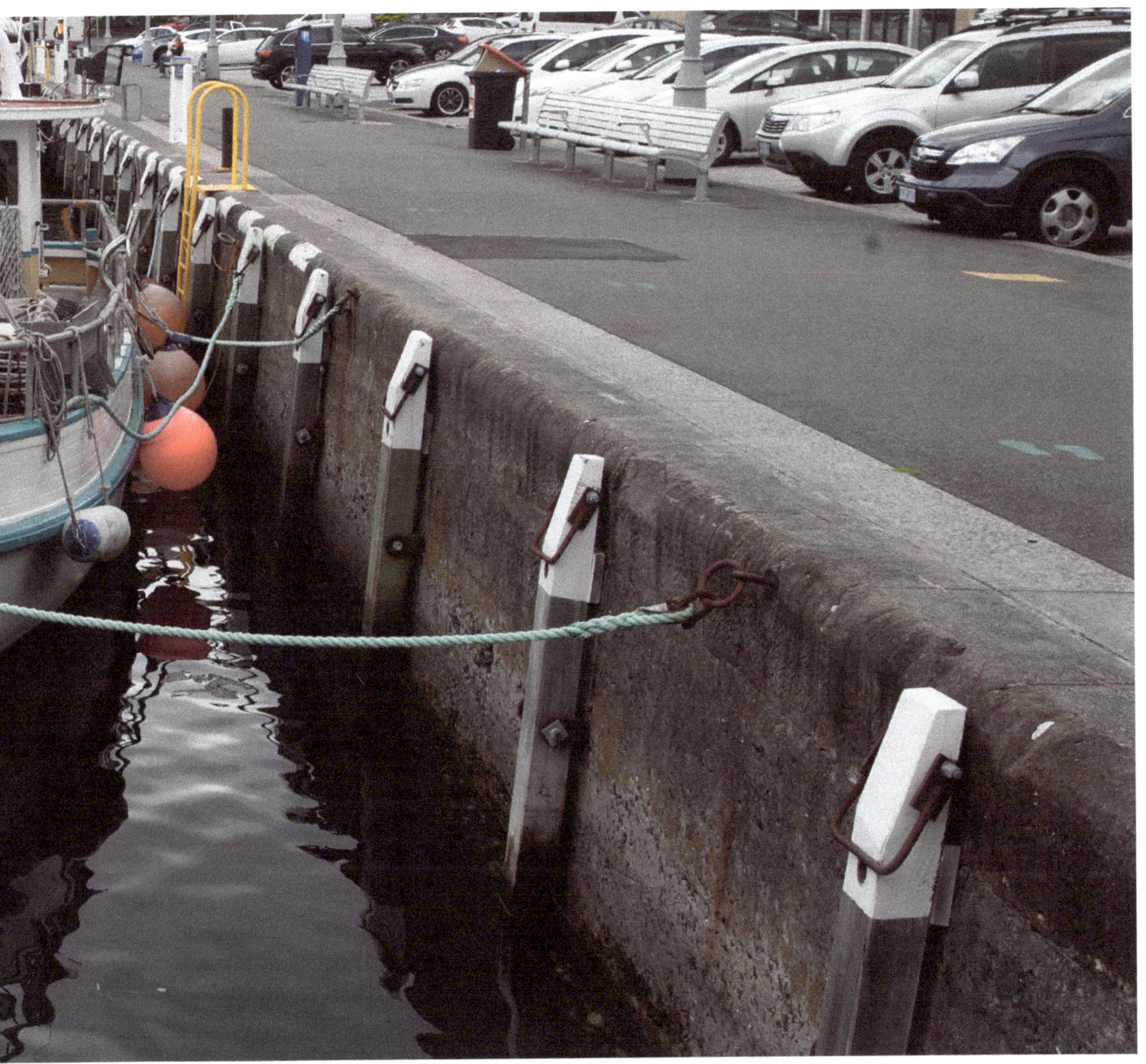

Crayfish Dip

SERVES 6-8 AS A STARTER

Crayfish dip is a luxurious treat, especially combined with the traditional flavours of tomato and Tabasco. You can buy cooked crayfish from your fishmonger, which makes this a very quick and easy recipe to whip up for a celebration.

1 crayfish

1 clove garlic

200 grams cream cheese

200ml mayonnaise (or aioli from page 90)

½ teaspoon Worcestershire sauce

2 tablespoons tomato sauce, chutney or relish

Tabasco sauce

To cook the crayfish, bring a saucepan of salted water to the boil, ensuring that it is large enough to submerge the crayfish. Add the crayfish, return the water to the boil and cook for 8 minutes. Meanwhile, fill the sink with iced water. After 8 minutes of cooking, remove the crayfish and plunge them into the sink of iced water for 10 minutes or until cool. Drain the crayfish. Remove all the meat from the fish, leaving some legs whole for a garnish. Chop the meat into 1cm cubes.

Using a food processor, blend the garlic, softened cream cheese, mayonnaise, and Worcestershire and tomato sauce. Add the Tabasco sauce to taste. In a bowl, gently fold the crayfish meat through the cream cheese mixture. Garnish with the crayfish legs and serve with fresh crusty bread, grissini or crackers.

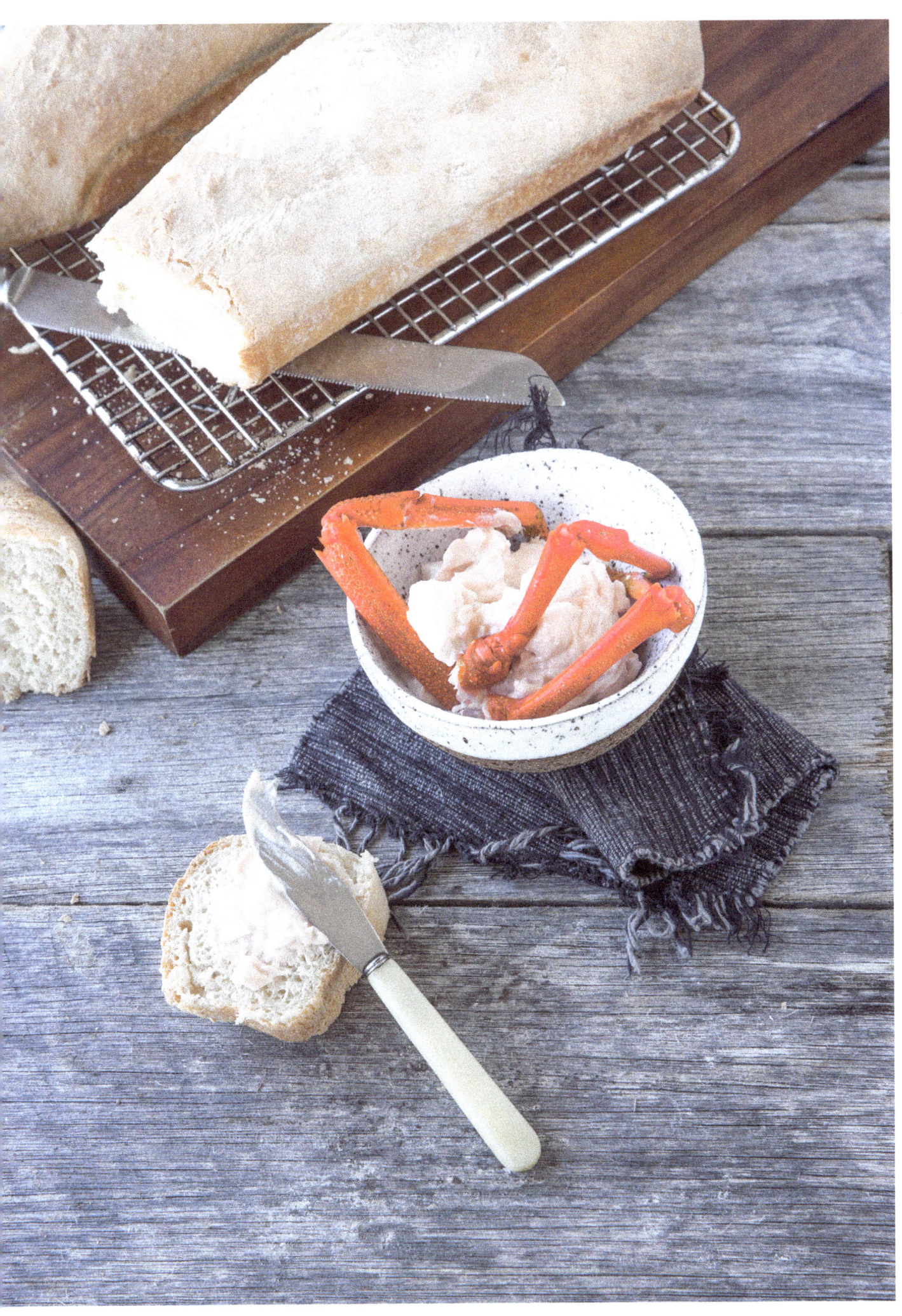

Crayfish with Smoked Cheddar Cheese Sauce

SERVES 2-4

Crayfish Mornay is a rich, indulgent treat. For a truly spectacular dish or a special occasion, you could use artisan cheese in the mornay sauce. One of my favourite cheeses to use here is Bruny Island Cheese's Tom, which is available here in Tasmania, but substitute your own favourite from a local cheesemaker.

2 crayfish

salt

SAUCE

40 grams butter

50 grams plain flour

400ml milk

salt and pepper

1 tablespoon parsley

100 grams smoked cheddar

60 grams parmesan cheese

To cook the crayfish, bring a large saucepan of salted water to the boil. Add the crayfish, return the water to the boil and cook for 8 minutes. Remove from the pot and drain. Cut the crayfish in half and remove the innards and intestinal tract. Remove the meat from the tail and chop into bite-sized cubes.

To make the sauce, melt the butter in a heavy-based saucepan over medium heat. Add the flour and cook stirring, for one minute. Stir in the milk, salt and pepper to taste, and bring to the boil stirring continuously, until the sauce thickens.

Finely chop the parsley and grate the cheddar and parmesan cheeses. Stir the parsley, parmesan cheese and 60g of cheddar cheese through the sauce. Stir the crayfish meat through the sauce and return to the shell. Sprinkle with the remaining cheddar cheese.

Heat the grill to medium/high heat and grill the crayfish for a couple of minutes, or until the cheese is melted and golden brown.

Serve immediately with fresh garden salad and potatoes.

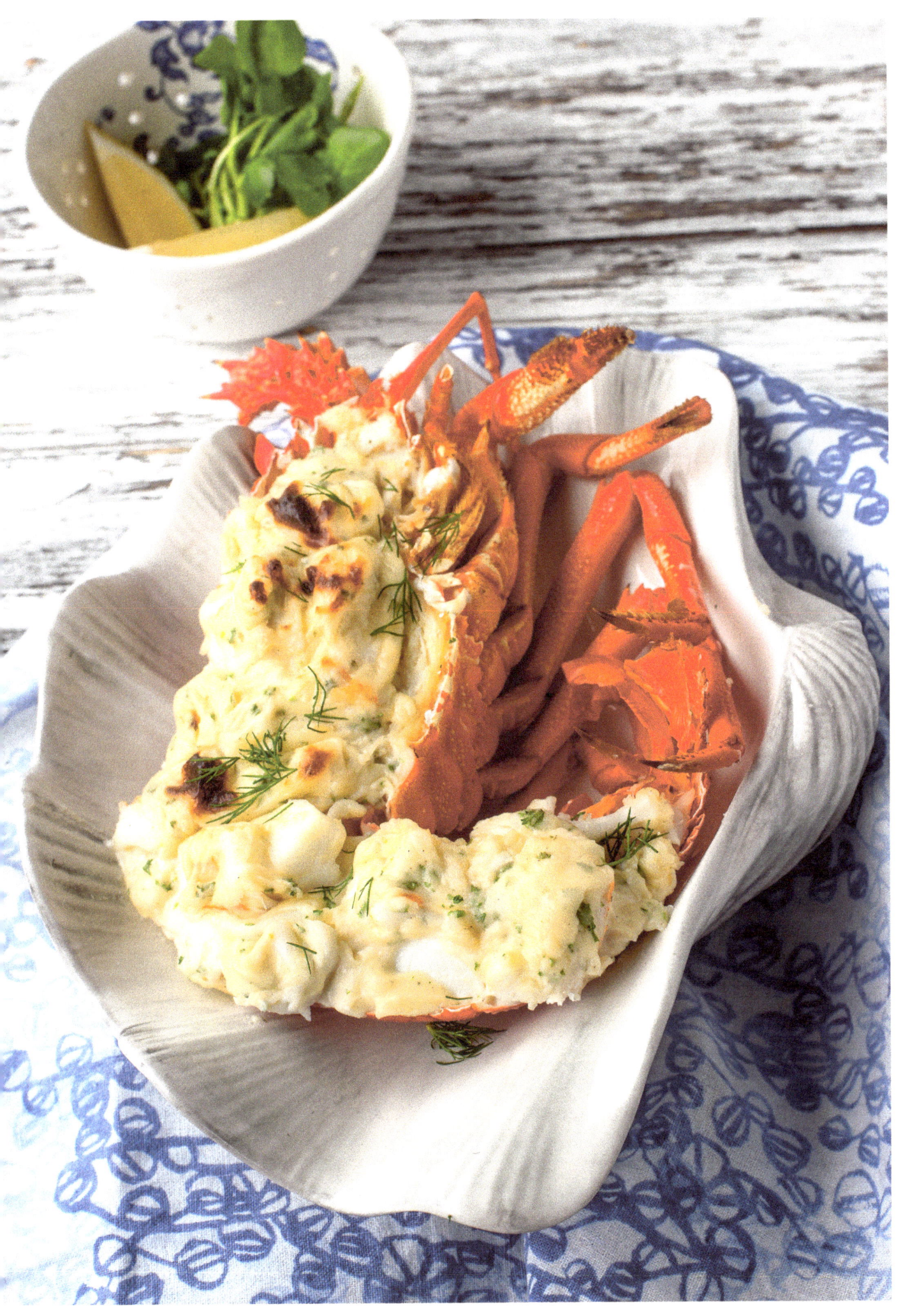

Crayfish with Homemade Cocktail Sauce

SERVES 2-4

2 whole crayfish

salt

COCKTAIL SAUCE

2 eggs

30ml white vinegar

1 clove garlic

salt and pepper

200ml extra virgin olive oil

2 tablespoons tomato sauce, tomato relish or chutney

1 teaspoon Worcestershire sauce

3 shakes Tabasco sauce (or to taste)

To cook the crayfish, bring a large saucepan of salted water to the boil. Add the crayfish, return the water to the boil and cook for 8 minutes. Meanwhile, fill the sink with iced water. Remove the crayfish from the saucepan and plunge into the iced water to stop the cooking process. Leave the crayfish in the iced water for 5-10 minutes to cool completely, and then drain.

To make the cocktail sauce, use a food processor to blend the eggs, vinegar, garlic and salt and pepper to taste. With the processor still running, slowly add the oil in a steady drizzle, until a thick, creamy emulsion has formed. Mix in the tomato, Worcestershire and Tabasco sauces.

Chop the crayfish to your liking, and serve with a crisp salad and the cocktail sauce.

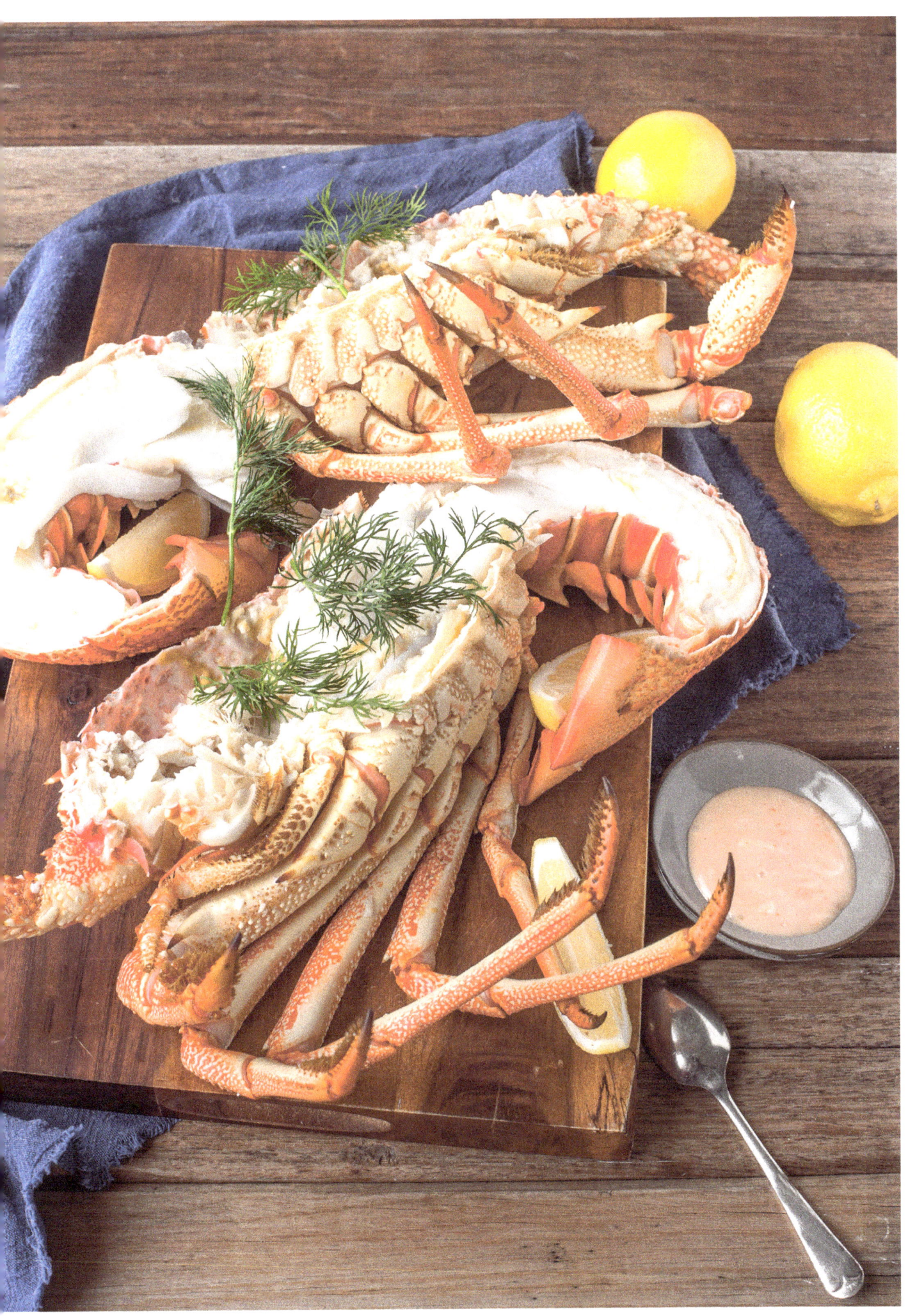

Crayfish with a Fennel Butter Sauce

SERVES 2-4

It is best to cook the crayfish as close to serving time as possible, so that the crayfish meat is still hot. You can start the fennel sauce the day before which gives the flavours more time to develop and intensify.

2 whole crayfish

salt

FENNEL BUTTER SAUCE

1 fennel bulb

½ onion

2 cloves garlic

1 leek

1 carrot

1 stick celery

100ml extra virgin olive oil

1 tablespoon fennel seed

100 grams plain flour

700ml chicken or vegetable stock

700ml cream

salt and pepper

100 grams butter

To cook the crayfish, bring a large saucepan of salted water to the boil. Add the crayfish, return the water to the boil and cook for 8 minutes. Remove from the pot and drain. Cut the crayfish in half, remove the meat from the tail and chop the meat into cubes.

To make the fennel sauce, roughly dice the fennel, onion, garlic, leek, carrot and celery. Heat the extra virgin olive oil in a heavy-based saucepan over medium heat, add the diced vegetables and fennel seed and sauté for a few minutes until softened.

Add the flour to the saucepan and cook stirring, for a few minutes. Add the stock, bring to the boil, reduce heat to a simmer and cook for 1 hour. This can be done a day ahead, to give more time for the flavors to develop. Add the cream, return to the boil and simmer for 15 minutes.

Season with salt and pepper and pour the sauce through a sieve to strain. Discard the solids, return the liquid to the saucepan. Whisk the cubed butter through the sauce.

Toss the pre-prepared crayfish meat through the sauce, and return the meat to the shell of the tail, with the remaining sauce poured over the top. Serve the crayfish with a crisp salad.

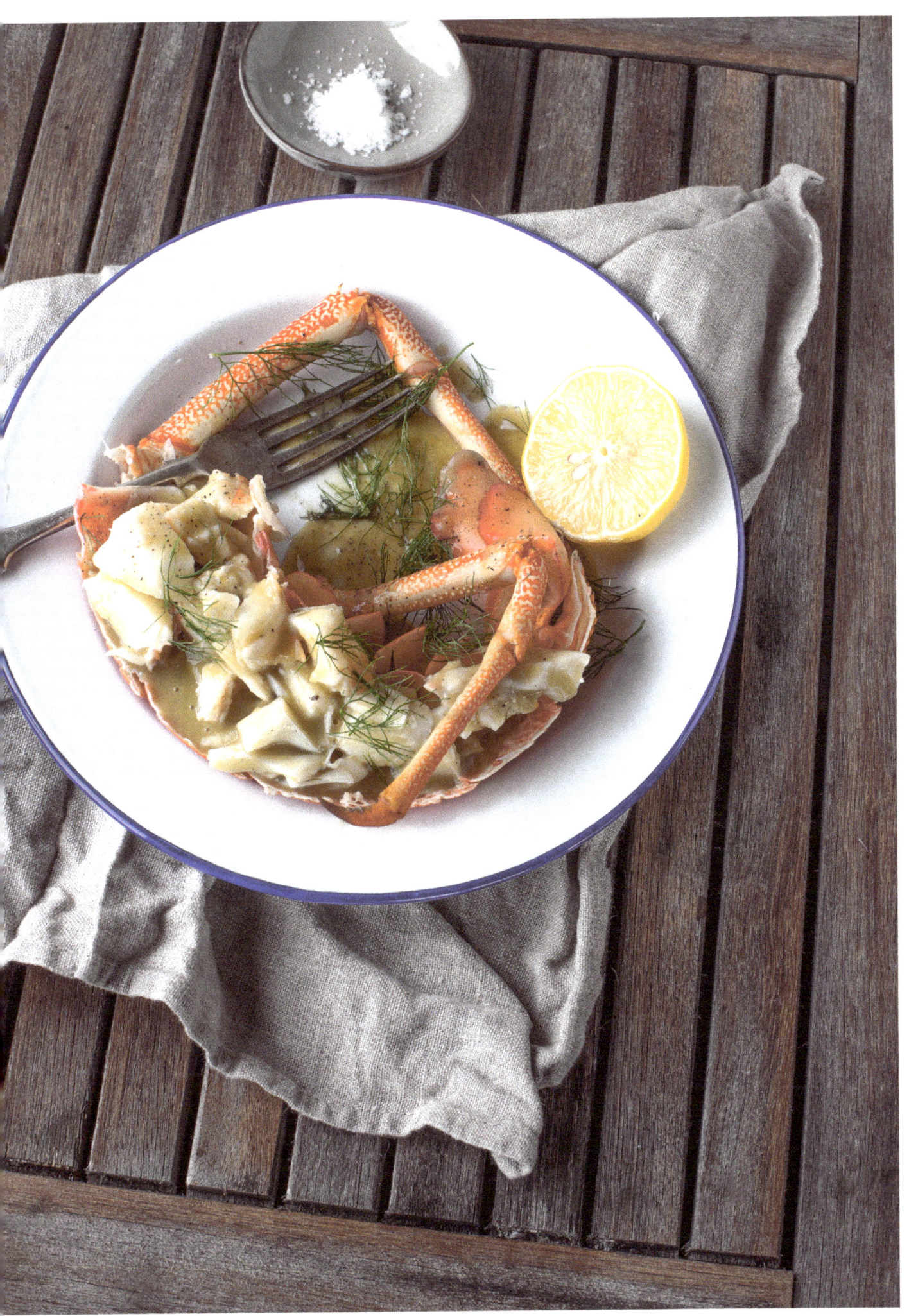

Crayfish with a Dill Hollandaise Sauce

SERVES 2-4

When making hollandaise sauce, the egg yolks need to be simultaneously whisked and lightly cooked. I find that the best way to do this without scrambling the eggs is over a pot of simmering water on the stovetop.

2 crayfish

salt

DILL HOLLANDAISE SAUCE

3 egg yolks

25ml white wine vinegar

150 grams butter

2 tablespoons dill

To cook the crayfish, bring a large saucepan of salted water to the boil. Add the crayfish, return the water to the boil and cook for 8 minutes. Meanwhile, fill the sink with iced water. Remove the crayfish from the saucepan and plunge into the iced water to stop the cooking process. Leave the crayfish in the iced water for 5-10 minutes to cool completely, and then drain. Cut the crayfish in half and remove the intestinal tract. Remove the meat, chop into cubes and return to the shell for serving.

To make the dill hollandaise sauce, place a heatproof bowl over a saucepan of simmering water. Add the egg yolks and vinegar to the bowl, and whisk until light and fluffy. Melt the butter and slowly drizzle into the egg mixture whilst whisking, to create a smooth, thick sauce. Stir through the finely chopped dill and season with salt and pepper.

Pour the hollandaise sauce over the cubed crayfish and serve with a crisp garden salad and freshly cooked pink-eye potatoes.

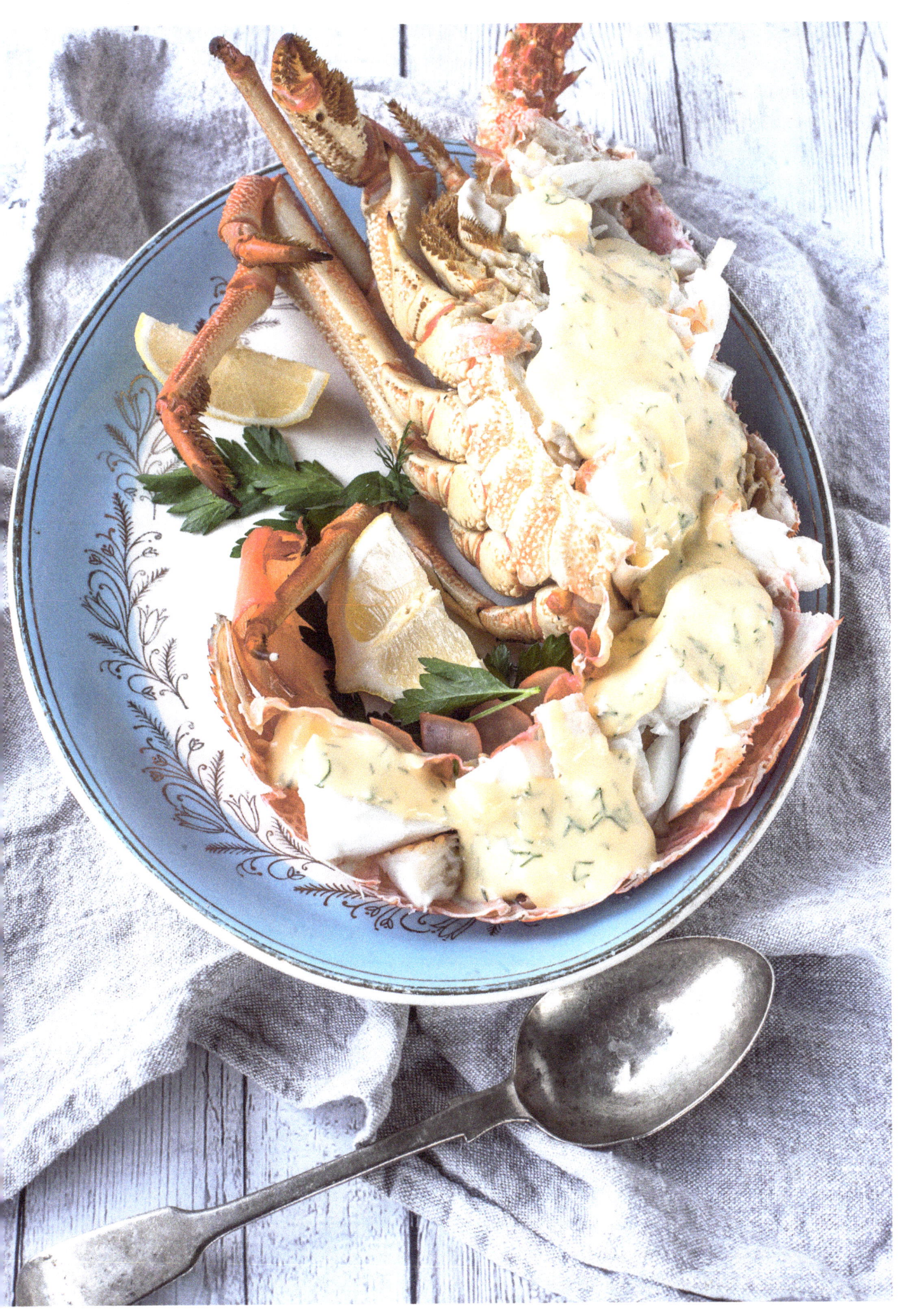

Barbequed Crayfish with Garlic Butter, Sage and Tarragon

SERVES 2-4

2 crayfish

GARLIC BUTTER

2 cloves garlic

1 tablespoon sage

1 tablespoon tarragon

100 grams butter

sea salt and cracked black pepper

To make the garlic butter, crush the garlic, finely chop the herbs and combine with the slightly softened butter, and salt and pepper to taste, mixing until well combined.

To prepare the crayfish, cut in half lengthways and remove all of the innards. Remove the crayfish meat from the shell, chop into cubes and return to the shell. Place spoonfuls of the butter mix on top of the crayfish, as well as gently pushing some butter in between the cubes of meat.

To cook the crayfish on the barbeque, pre-heat to low, and barbeque for approximately 15 minutes with the lid shut. To cook in the oven, pre-heat to 180°C, place crayfish on a baking tray and cook for 15 minutes, or until the meat is cooked through. The crayfish is delicious served with boiled, new-season, pink-eye potatoes rolled in garlic butter leftover from the crayfish.

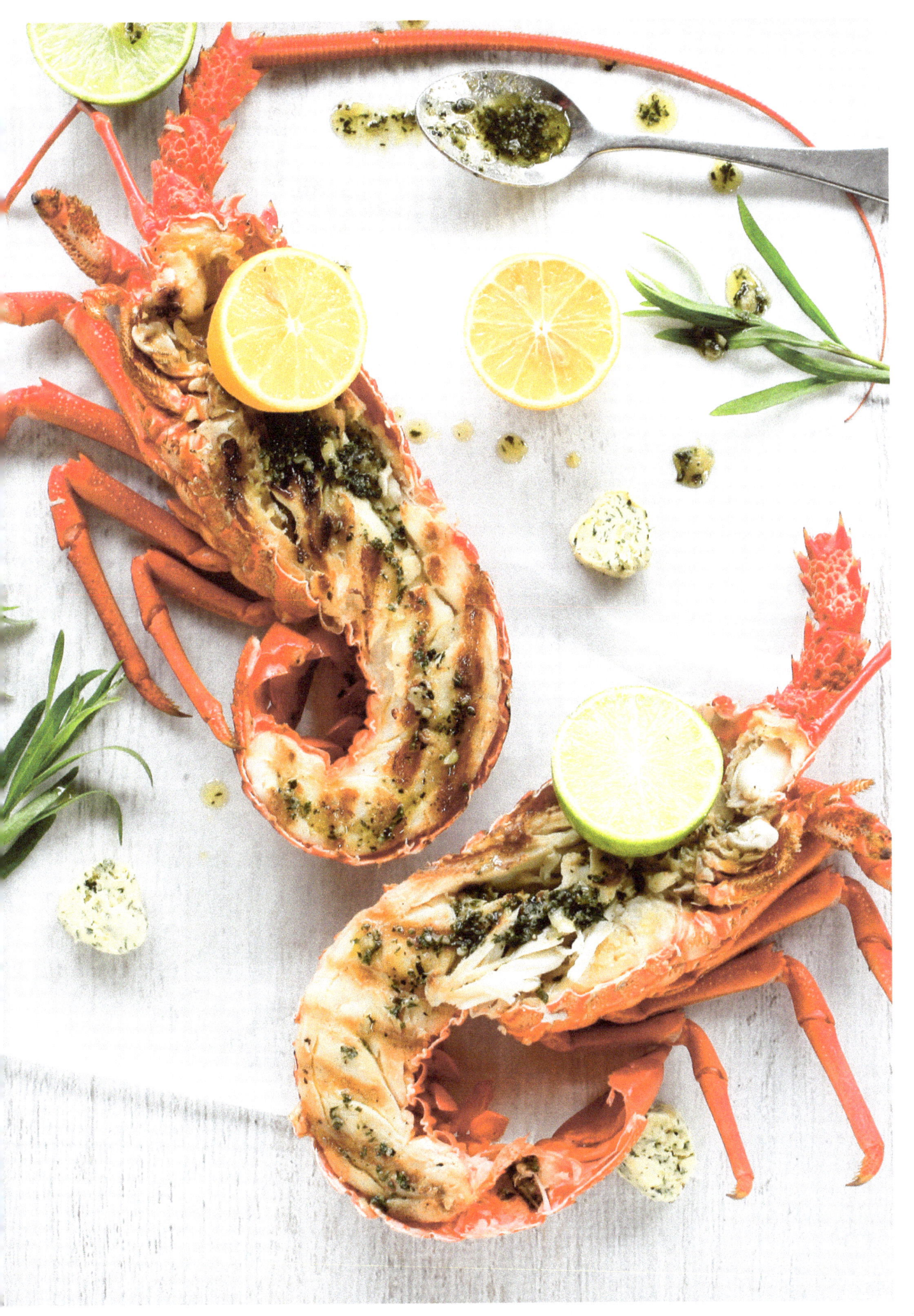

INDEX

A
Abalone with a Lime, Watercress and Goats Cheese Salad 36

B
Baked Fish with a Gremolata Crust, Caper Potato Mash and Lemon Butter 112
Baked Salmon with Pumpkin Pancakes, Crispy Bacon and Honey Mustard Aioli 128
Barbequed Crayfish with Garlic Butter, Sage and Tarragon 148
Barbequed Octopus with Feta Risotto Balls and Lemon Aioli 98
Barbequed Octopus with Pea, Cabbage and Feta Salad 96
Beer Battered Fish 86
Black Lip Mussels in a White Wine, Caper, Prosciutto, Tomato Cream Sauce with Spinach Fettuccini 30

C
Caper Tart with Smoked Salmon and Red Onion Jam 54
Chilli Mussels with Spaghetti, Chorizo and Tomato Sauce 32
Chilli Salted Fish with Spring Vegetable Risotto 110
Crayfish Dip 138
Crayfish with a Dill Hollandaise Sauce 146
Crayfish with a Fennel Butter Sauce 144
Crayfish with Homemade Cocktail Sauce 142
Crayfish with Smoked Cheddar Cheese Sauce 140

D
Dill and Feta Omelette 58

F
Family Salmon Casserole 52
Fish and Potato Croquettes 82
Fish Baked with Tomato, Garlic and Lemon with Homemade Gnocchi 116
Fish Burgers 74
Fish Chowder 66
Fish Lasagna with Fennel and Tarragon 68
Fish Pie 70
Fish with a Zucchini Salad 130
Fish with Peas and Burnt Butter 132
Five Spice Poached Coconut Salmon 126

INDEX

G
Garlic Buttered Scallops on Fillet Steak with Hollandaise ... 24
Gnocchi in Cream Sauce with Salmon ... 44
Grilled Octopus with Spinach and Cheese Pie ... 104

H
Honey Soy Marinated Fish and Noodle Salad ... 80

L
Laksa ... 62
Lemon and Oregano Fish with Fresh Burghul Salad ... 108

M
Macadamia Crusted Fish with Wasabi Potato Mash and Beetroot and Lime Chutney ... 122
Moroccan Seafood Stew ... 72
Mussels in Dill and Coconut Curry with Rice Noodles ... 26
Mussels with Pumpkin Ravioli, Brown Butter and Asparagus ... 28

N
Natural Oysters with Lemon and Parsley Vinaigrette ... 19

O
Oysters Florentine ... 12
Oysters Grilled with Prosciutto and Gruyere ... 14
Oysters Topped with Red Wine Vinegar, Capers and Gherkin ... 18
Oysters Topped with Smoked Salmon and Creme Fraiche ... 16
Oysters Topped with Tomato, Tabasco and Vodka Salsa ... 15

P
Pan-Fried Fish with a Blue Cheese and Potato Gratin and Cauliflower Puree ... 120
Panko Crumbed Abalone ... 34
Peppered Tuna Steak with a Warm Marinated Vegetable Salad and Grilled Kefalograviera Cheese ... 118
Pickled Octopus with a Greek Style Salad ... 102
Pink Eye Potato and Salmon Salad ... 46

INDEX

S

Salmon and White Bean Salad … 50
Salmon Omlette … 40
Salmon Poached in a Thyme and Mushroom Cream Sauce … 124
Salmon Rashers with French Toast and Maple Syrup … 56
Salt and Sichuan Peppered Oysters … 10
Salt and Sichuan Peppered Squid with Lemon Aioli … 92
Scallops Wrapped in Bacon with Spicy Tomato Sauce … 22
Seafood Risotto … 78
Smoked Salmon Pizza with Capers, Red Onion and Sour Cream … 42
Soy and Balsamic Marinated Fish … 114
Spicy Fish Tortillas … 64
Spring Rolls … 84
Squid Spaghetti with Lemon and Garlic … 100
Stuffed Squid with Red Pepper Sauce … 94

T

Tempura Oysters with Asian Dipping Sauce … 20
Tomato and Tarragon Seafood Broth … 76
Tuna Carpaccio … 134
Tuna Nori Rolls … 48

W

Whole Baked Fish with Feta, Roast Bintje Potatoes, Spinach and Skordallia … 88

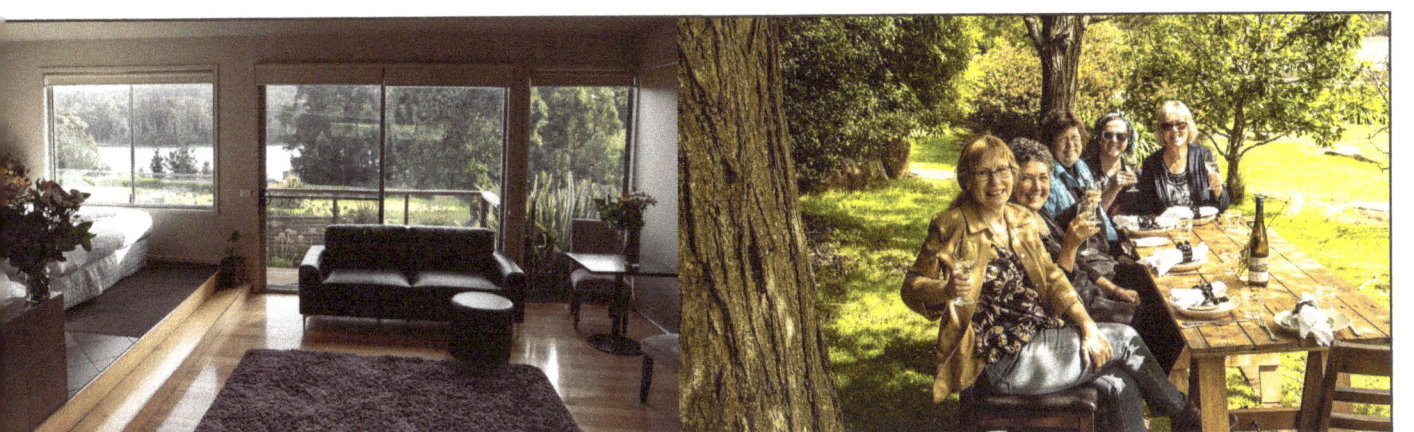

Little Norfolk Bay
EVENTS & CHALETS

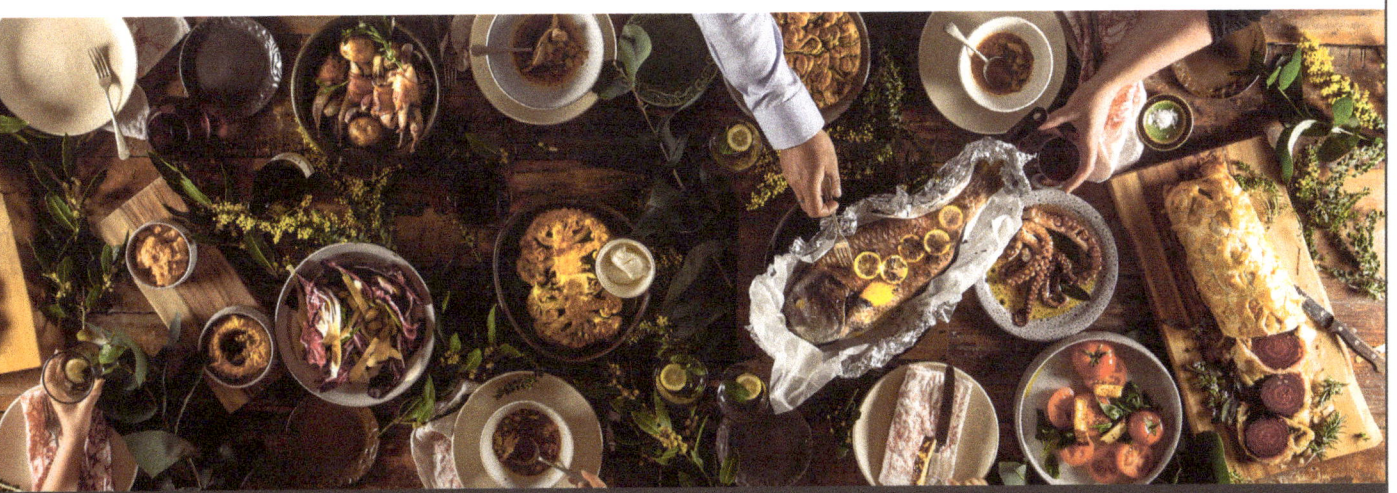

Accommodation, Cooking Retreats, Workshops and Indulgence Weekends in Taranna on the gorgeous Tasman Peninsula. Perfect for corporate or private gatherings and celebrations. Contact Chef and Host Eloise Emmett to design your unique experience.

www.eloiseemmett.com
www.littlenorfolkbayeventsandchalets.com

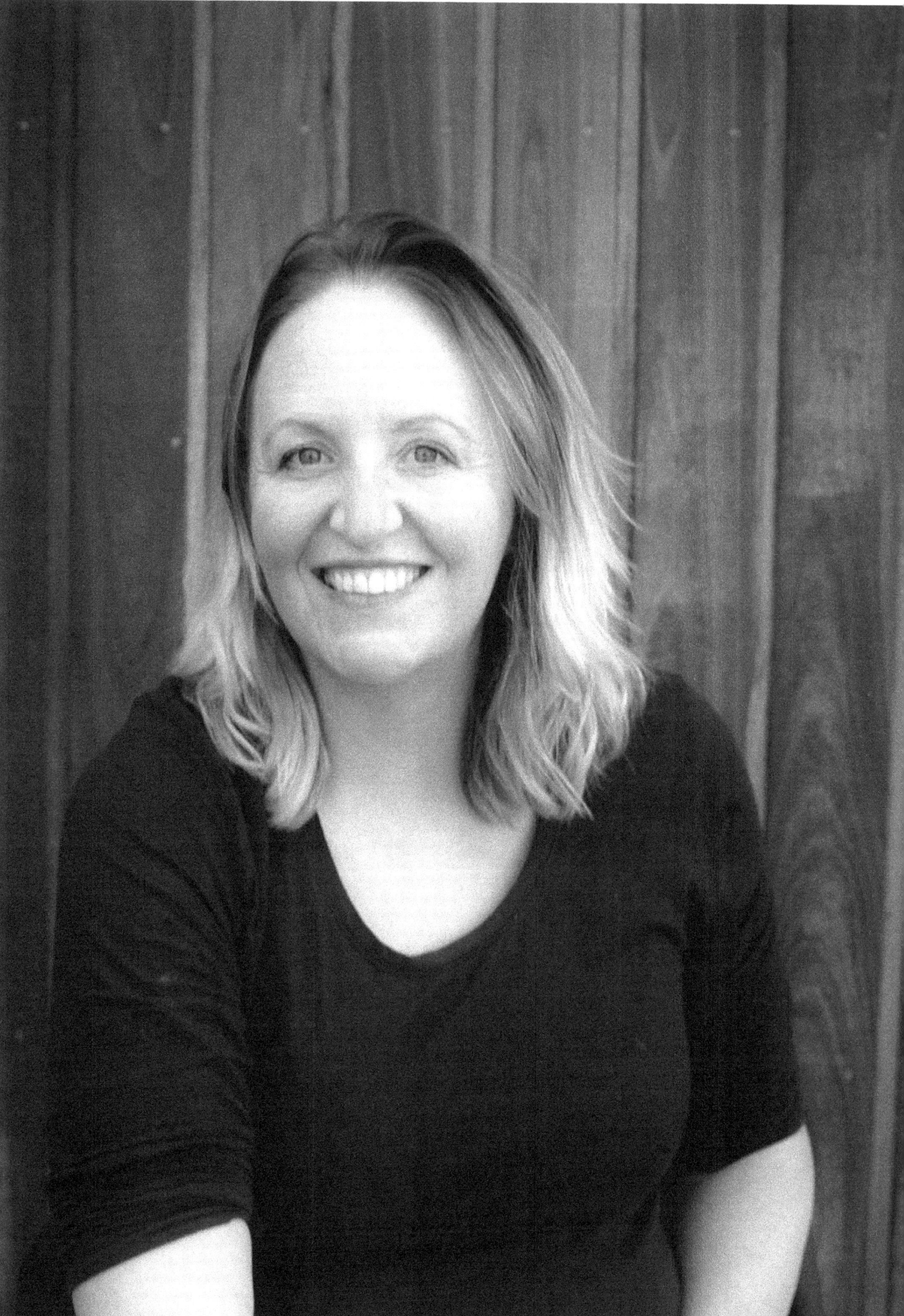

About the Author

Eloise Emmett is a Trade Qualified Chef with nearly 30 years experience in commercial kitchens, including 7 years as the Chef and owner of her own popular restaurant The Mussel Boys on the Tasman Peninsula. She now hosts weekend cooking retreats and indulgence weekends at Little Norfolk Bay Events and Chalets, which is a luxury accommodation retreat and boutique cooking school.

Eloise has been writing and photographing recipes for her popular website eloiseemmett.com since 2012. In 2013 Eloise co-authored the *Bream Creek Farmers Market Cookbook*, in 2015 she published *The Real Food for Kids Cookbook* and in 2016 she published the multi award winning *Seafood Everyday*. *Seafood Everyday* won **Best Fish and Seafood Book in Australia**, and **Best Book by a Woman Chef in Australia**. It then went on to become the third best seafood cookbook in the world, when it and won third place in **The Best Fish and Seafood** category at the **Gourmand World Cookbook Awards**. In 2017 Eloise published the first print of *The Tasmania Pantry* and in 2020 she published the second edition, *The Tasmania Pantry 2*.

Eloise loves cooking, styling and photographing food and shopping for props at op-shops and markets. She has three children and with her fisherman husband and they live on the stunning Tasman Peninsula in Tasmania. Most of all Eloise loves educating families about how important cooking, preparing meals and eating real food. Her core message, is that cooking is not hard and is a lot more economical way to feed your family, and she encourages even the busiest families to prepare easy meals from real food.

www.eloiseemmett.com

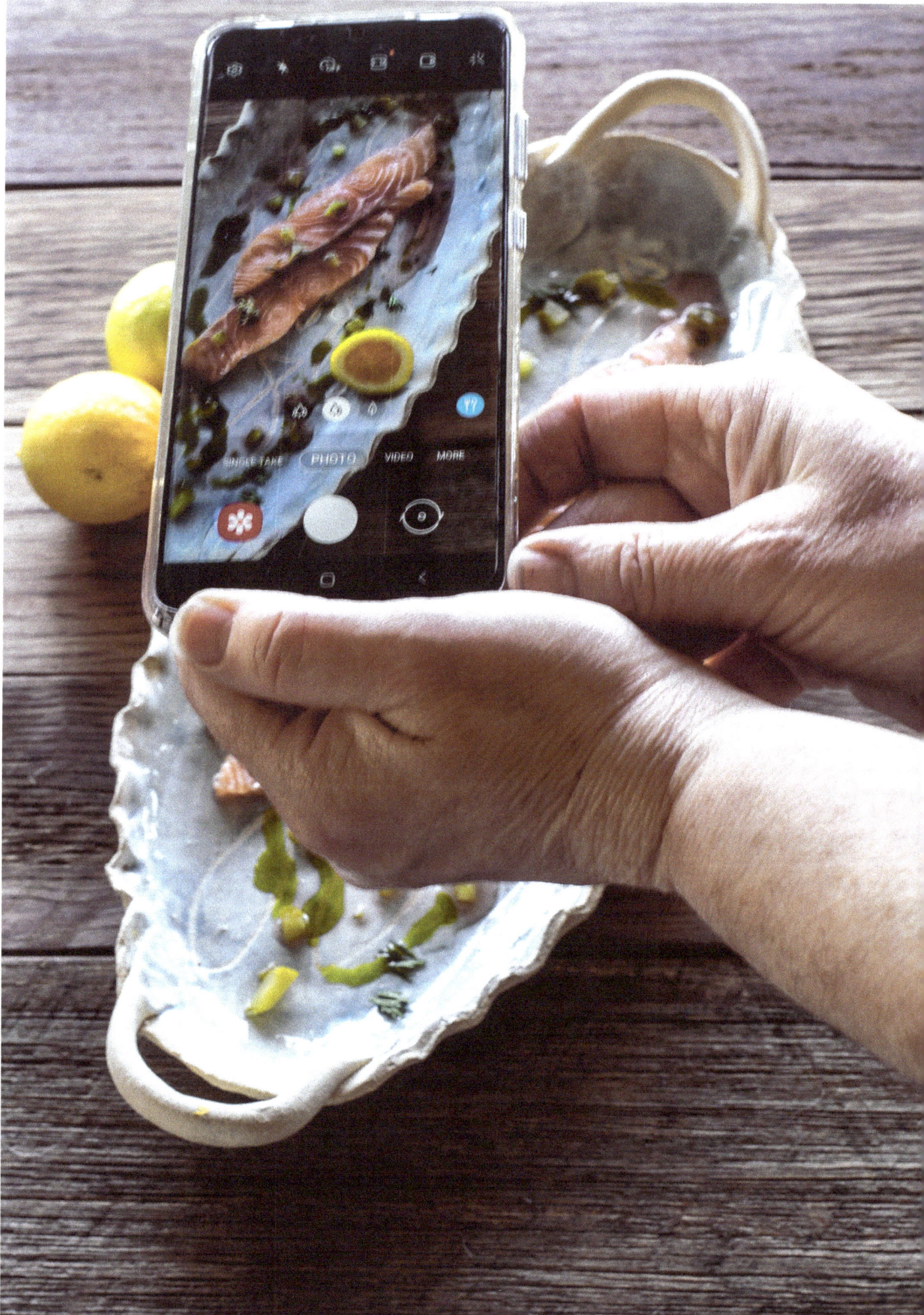

Feeling inspired?
Would you like to learn more?

You might enjoy my many in person and online workshops!

I cover many basics such as:

Seafood Cooking

Bread Making

Photography

Party Planning

Self Publishing

Phone Photography and Food Styling

Please find more information
at www.eloiseemmett.com

Eloise Emmett

CHEF PHOTOGRAPHER STYLIST

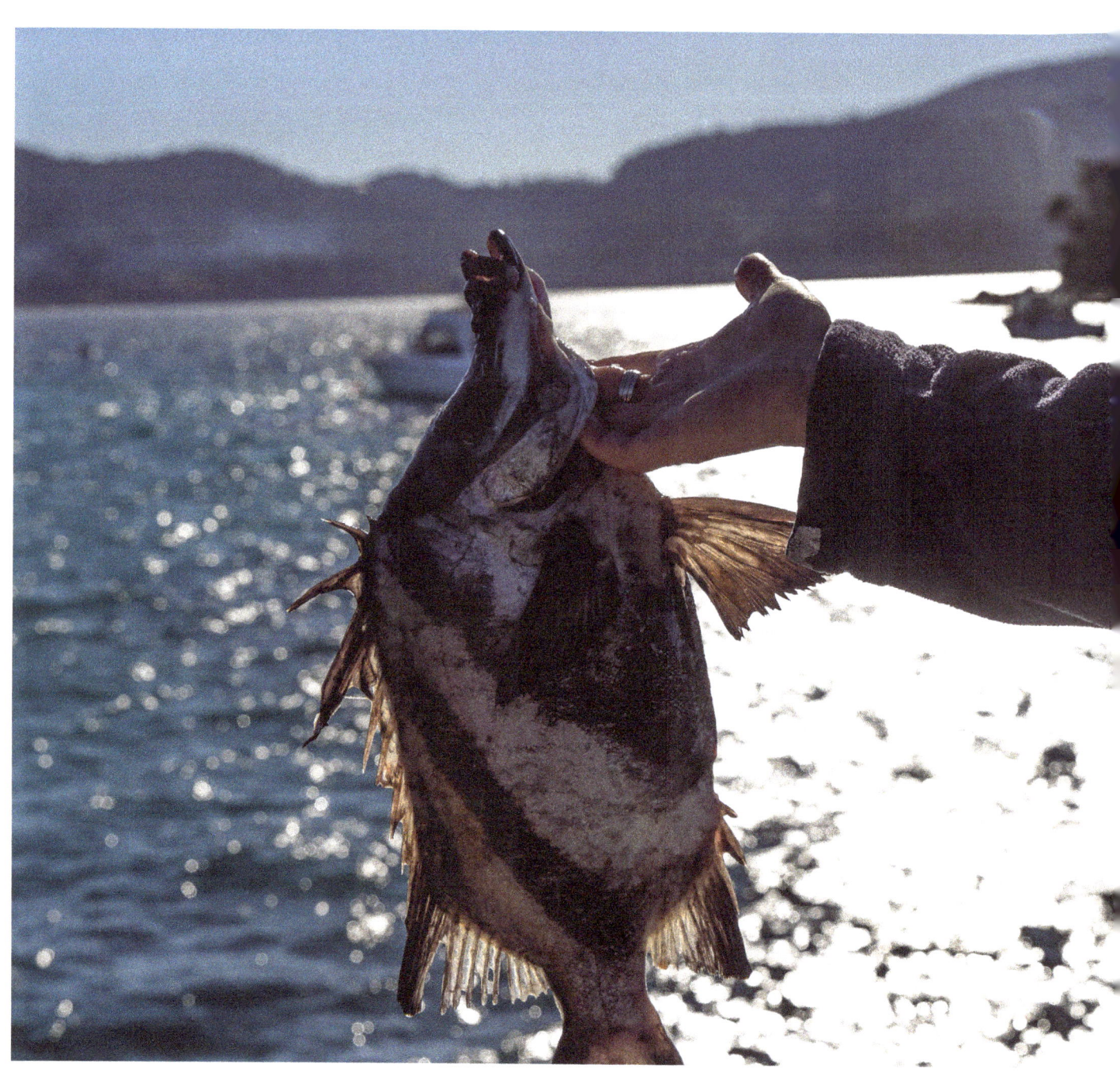

www.ingramcontent.com/pod-product-compliance
Lightning Source LLC
Chambersburg PA
CBHW041036020526
44118CB00043BA/2998